Starving to be Fat

Marco Girgenti

Copyright 2009 by Marco Girgenti

All rights reserved

No part of this book may be reproduced, stored in a retrieval system, or transmitted by any means, electronic, mechanical, photocopying, recording, or otherwise, without written permission from the author or publisher. There is one exception. Brief passages may be quoted in articles or reviews.

Library and Archives Canada Cataloguing in Publication

Cataloguing data available through Library and Archives Canada

ISBN 978-1-926582-25-2

Dedications and Acknowledgements for "Starving to be Fat".

For my son, Anthony. My hero.

For my mom, the strongest woman I know, and for my dad, I know you can see me. See? I turned out okay after all!

For Susan, the love of my life. Thank you for your beauty on all levels, your love and faith in me, and for your companionship and devotion. I love you. You are a true champion. "Poise and power," indeed.

For my extended family, Mauro, Connie, Laura, Deborah and Sarah

For David Appia, a friend who has stayed with me in places where lesser men may have not. You are a creative marvel, and your day is coming.

For Alex Portelli and Kenneth Nail, aka my own dream team. Three words: wisdom, faith and courage. Without you, this book would still be just a bunch of diary notes. Thank you for believing in me.

Finally, and most importantly, to my God, who always leads us in triumph.

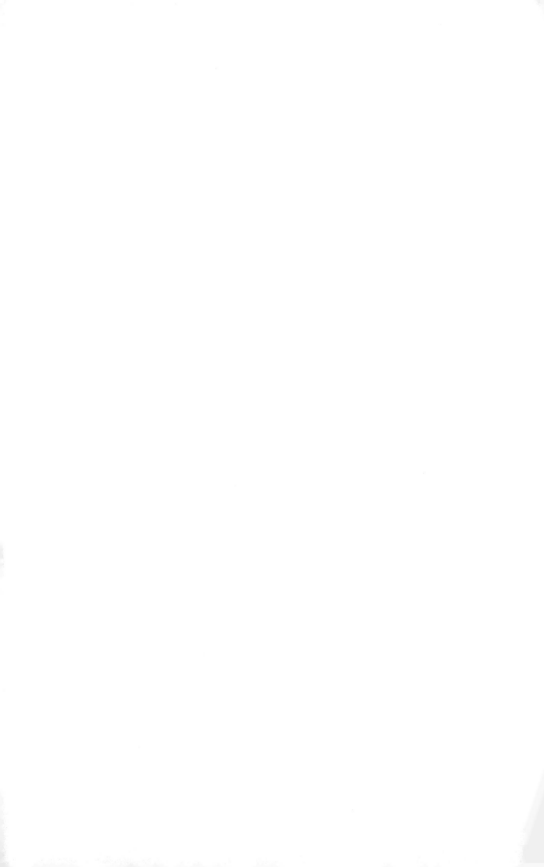

Table of Contents

Preface	7
Diary of a Fat Man	9
Image and Images	15
Fat Has Lousy Aim	19
My Friend Eats Anything She Wants...	23
A Simple Plan	27
Easy Does It	31
Food Or Faux?	35
Calorie Confusion	39
Live and Let Die	43
Failing To Plan	49
Decisions, Decisions	51
Horror Stories and Misconceptions from my Life as a Consultant	56
Move!	63
Starving to be Fat	67
Susan, the Last Thing I Ever Expected	71
"Poise and Power" a chapter by Susan Braumberger-Arruda. National Figure Champion.	75
Small Changes, Big Results	85
What's Eating You?	89
Yesterday, Malnutrition Seemed So Far Away...	93
Trainers. Certified or Certifiable?	99
Final Thoughts	105

Preface

"My name is Marco and I am 41-years-old. My sister died when I was ten, my father died when I was 17, I got married, divorced 13 years later, and now have a teenage boy in my full-time care who is autistic. Along the way I lost 140 lbs. (that was six years ago) and it has never returned. In August of 2007, I became the top fitness consultant for a major fitness company. I am also practically engaged to a national fitness figure model champion."

Applause followed.

That was my opening statement at a board meeting with the heads of a major fitness company.

Life will never be devoid of challenges, we might as well make peace with that war right now.

I hated fat, but it loved me; it was my best friend as well as my arch enemy. No truer case of Jekyll and Hyde could be found. Fat would always be there to comfort me, but then later to torment me. While I could not control people dying around me or my son's autism, I **could** control food. It was the worst type of control to have. You see, even though I was abusing my body, I was **in control** of what I was doing to myself. No one controlled me or forced me to become overweight, it was all me and I had no one controlling me, but myself. I know, it sounds ridiculous and it certainly was a poor approach. One could call it a form of negative or destructive control to dealing with problems. I could control overeating and it was within my power to decide to eat cartons of ice cream and boxes of cookies or chips, or not. At least I **thought** I could control it, but in the end it wound up controlling me.

People overeat for different reasons. As a fitness consultant I met with thousands of people. While each of them had a different story the outcome was in large part the same in each case; people became stressed, depressed, and then ate themselves to hundreds of pounds of excess weight. From anorexics to gastric bypass patients, diabetics, cancer survivors, and 13 year olds weighing in at over 300 lb., all of them used food in some way to help them deal with their problems. I sat in my office searching for a way to help each of them.

Fat kills, but it kills a lot more than just our bodies; it assassinates our self-esteem. I know this first hand as the toll my extra weight took on me still reaches out to me from the grave in an attempt to once again be my "friend." I know I will never gain that weight back since I have changed my lifestyle completely. I have kept that weight off for over eight years now and reduced my pant size from 56 to 36, but the mental aspect of that fat battle continues years later, even after slaying that "Goliath."

How did I do it? Am I smarter than you, gracious reader? Probably not, but chances are that you are reading this book because you are searching for a way out of fat and into control of your life and health. If that is indeed your quest, then I think aspects of my story could help to inspire and equip you to reach that goal.

Take it from a man who could not get the seatbelt around his waist on a flight to New York City years ago—fat **is** defeatable!

Who holds the story of my struggle and victory in their hands? Who is reading my book? Are you a millionaire or a professor? Perhaps you are a caretaker, housewife, or nurse? Maybe you are a teenager? What you do for a living has nothing to do with this. No amount of money, no weight loss guru, not a single person on earth can win this battle for you, only **you** can do that. You **have** the power within you to take control of your life or to fail completely.

I had to come to that harsh realization myself; it was MY fault and no one else's that I got fat and only I could change that.

This book is not about quick fixes, nor is it a diet or exercise book. This book **is** about baby steps that turned into giant leaps of victory. It is not the "Marco" system of fat loss. Rather, this book is about common sense and how an everyday guy turned the tables on depression, low self-esteem, and fat.

I dare you to step out in faith, practical common sense and take down the enemy that has bullied and ridiculed you for years. Enough is enough! Do you want to fail, yet again? Do you want to yo-yo up and down with your weight? Or are you ready for a new way of living, a new way of feeling about yourself and, yes, a new wardrobe?

If you have the courage to believe you can win this war, then I implore you to keep reading. If you do not think you have that courage, this book might just help you find it.

"Diary of a Fat Man"

(excerpts from the beginning of and during my weight loss journey)

"Sir, can you move please? You are too fat to sit here."

That statement pierced my heart and it was also the first time I realized just how out of control my weight was. Within the 24 hours after hearing those words, I had landed in New York City for a dressed rehearsal for a musical I was conducting. I donned my tux and thought: "Wow, black is slimming." As the curtain rose I was momentarily distracted while I reflected on the road my musical partner and I travelled to finally reach New York. Some of the score papers on my stand had fallen off and I bent over to pick them up. The next sound that could be heard was not the opening strains of the overture, but, instead, the sound went something like "rrrrrrrrrrrip," as my size 56 pants tore from stem to stern in front of the 150 people sitting behind me. I wrapped my tux jacket around my waist and ran out of the room, embarrassed and crying. I was devastated.

October 30, 1995

Dear diary...Everyone is looking at me, I can feel it. Anytime I find the courage to actually go to a party or out with friends, I know I'll be the fattest one in the room. Look at me, who would want to date someone that looks like me? Heck, I can't even bend over to tie my shoes, much less go out. I really need to go on a diet. That's it, I am cutting carbs and fats. Salads are the way to go, yeah, that's what I'll do. Gonna buy some of those shakes, too— especially the low carb ones. Wow look, they've got amazing flavours and they are SO low calorie! I do not care if I have to starve myself, I'll do anything. ANYTHING, is better than this.

Every time I go buy clothes, I can't shop where "others" do. I need a "special" shop; one that carries my size. The clothes are so expensive and forget about wearing the latest fashions. It's not that I expect to look like a super-model, I just wish I could at least look better, feel better, and be healthier. Not just for me, but for my son and the rest of my family as well.

The are no pictures of me in my home. As a matter of fact, very few pictures of me exist at all. Why, you may ask? Simply because I don't want to look at myself, not in the mirror and certainly not in a picture with all my friends who are so much fitter, slimmer, and healthier than I am. Who needs a constant reminder of what a sorry case I am?

Right now I have no self-esteem and I hate myself. I am doomed. It seems I will never lose this weight. Some of my friends have tried to lose weight and nothing has worked for them either. Not the diets or the gym. The tapes, the "infomercial walker," or miracle ab-crunchers "only available on TV" they bought, well, their laundry looks great hanging from it.

Why should I even bother trying to do this? It's odd. People look at me and see me as successful. I make good money, am a doting father, an accomplished musician... but the first thing they think? "He's fat." Automatically they assume I cannot control myself. Boy, people can sure be harsh. ***The problem is that they're right and that fact alone hurts me all the more. At this rate, I will be dead by my mid-30's.***

The excerpt above exposes me at my weakest and lowest. Fat loss seemed impossible! I had yet to embark on research that would arm me with the proper approach and prove me wrong. I went through what most people do. I was looking for the "magic bullet," the quick fix. I was willing to spend as much money as I needed to in order to lose weight. I did not at this point understand that "weight" was a lot more than just pounds of fat and that the "good" weight I had (the lean mass), needed to be not only preserved, but also increased. My following journal entry takes place four years later, after spending that time researching what my approach should be.

December 3, 1999

*For three weeks now, I have driven to the local gym. I drove up to the front door and just sat there for a few minutes, thinking. The gym was a no go; I drove off and went to the coffee shop instead. Why am I so **afraid** of walking in there? Are there any other* *fat people in there or is everyone in perfect shape? Will they even allow a fat guy to have a membership there?* **Everyone** *is going to look at me. "Wow, look at the fat guy." I can already hear it!*

Yes, I was petrified by the fear of even walking in there! My first day was very difficult for me, both emotionally and physically. There were too many mirrors in the gym for my liking. I was all sweaty when I was done and yet I did not even have the courage to shower in the men's change room. Yes, I would have much rather smelled bad than look bad.

January 1, 2000

Well, today I started my workout! A few light weights and attempted five minutes on the treadmill, but I only lasted three. I threw up all over myself and the treadmill and ran out of the gym. Keep looking in the mirror, Marco. Keep thinking "who would find this blob of fat attractive? Who would want to be with someone who looks like this? Think of the nice clothes, looking good and feeling strong, feeling in control and sex appeal.

Never stop! GREATNESS at any cost!

January 3, 2000

Second day. Pain everywhere yesterday! I could not get up to take my son to school. Did I overdo it? Or am I so brutally out of shape that this is the natural result of actually moving! I tried to walk on the treadmill again today and again, I threw up after three minutes. Seems like if my fat won't kill me, then trying to get in shape certainly will! I am feeling a lot more energetic though and I am looking forward to tomorrow. At least I am TRYING. Remember how good you feel after working out first thing in the morning. "Bed or workout?" I feel bagged in the morning after dropping Anthony off at school. Just remember how good you felt doing it even though you were tired.

All for now.

February 3, 2000

Oh YES, I am feeling great! Arm muscles are starting to show! I did 22 minutes on the treadmill. I can't believe I got here after having thrown up my first two days. I have learened that small steps work best for me. The best thing I did was to try to add just one minute per week to my treadmill time. I did make a mistake though; I changed my breakfast and had milk (with the rest of my food). I decided to try a citrus flavoured drink during my treadmill time. The two ingredients did not like each other at all and I wound up vomiting again! I have no pain or soreness today. I dropped the amount of weight I was lifting in order to maintain proper form. I am feeling awesome and am having to take afternoon naps. The two days off over the weekend were a mistake, I think they cost me in the endurance and strength areas. I hope I can get to the gym five days per week soon! Remember to establish an exercise program before leaving for New York City.

FINALLY, someone NOTICED! Two of my friends (who didn't even know I had been going to the gym) both said I looked like I'd lost weight! When they said this, I instantly became emotional and cried right on the spot in front of them.

MOTIVATED? Oh yeah! But still, a VERY long road ahead of me.

NEVER STOP! I Like it when people notice that I've lost weight instead of what they used to say about me.

End of entry.

I came back from New York City after six weeks and was a staggering 30 lb. lighter! What I had lost was a lot of water weight (water that had been stored in my body for years, due to dehydration) as well as fat and probably some muscle as well. All I knew was that I felt a lot different and that the pants I had bought one month earlier no longer fit me.

I continued to journal my beginnings for about two months and then stopped. I was over the toughest hump—the beginning! The next time I had cause to write in my diary was years later, after my marriage had ended. In the meantime, Anthony had been born and had been diagnosed with autism, a whole other type of challenge for me to face!

In 2006, I passed the Personal Trainer Specialist certification exam! A few weeks later, I was hired as a personal trainer for a major fitness company. When I received my name tag and uniform shirt, I ran to the car and cried like a baby. I went home and had what I can only describe as my Jerry Maguire moment! I wrote an email to the staff of the gym entitled "It's not a shirt, it's a badge!"

There are still moments now that I see myself in the mirror as I demonstrate exercises to new people at the gym where I work. I see my reflection, leaner and stronger and my soul smiles on the inside of me and says...
   ..."**you did it Marco. You really did it!**"
SO CAN YOU!

Image and Images

Images are powerful things; and their primary use in the corporate world and media is to embed a picture in our minds that instantly causes us to associate or think about a particular product, idea or company. If I were a betting man, I'd wager that there are at least five logos within eye shot of where you are sitting right now and if there aren't five I'd bet you can **think** of ten just off the top of your head.

IMAGES IN OUR CULTURE

An image is so powerful; it can define an entire industry. I'll have to qualify that statement here: all you have to do is think of the famous Nike "swoosh" to understand what I mean. Images, however, are more than just mere company logos. All of you in your teens and early twenties, who are reading this book, lend me your ears and imaginations. Think of two of your favourite singers, these could be R&B, Rap, Hip-Hop, Pop, Dance, etc. Think of some of the album covers and videos featuring these singers....Got that picture in your mind's eye? Okay, now imagine these singers as considerably overweight, would you still like them as much as you do now, even without their cut, super hot bods? You might quickly say yes since you are into them for their "music." I was in the music business for a living professionally for 15 years and I can tell you from experience that if you are overweight or you don't conform to a certain ideal or look, that you are going to have an uphill battle with your record label. Now, I understand that it is pleasing to watch someone who is attractive to you, but years ago it just didn't matter as much as it does today.

There is a songwriter named Christopher Cross who in the 80's wrote some of the most beautiful adult contemporary music I had ever heard. Christopher reached global fame with his hit song called "Sailing", as well as others. He sings very well and is an extremely good guitarist, but Christopher does not have movie star looks or a body to match, by his own admission. As musically brilliant as he is, he vanished off the pop charts very quickly even though his hits were covered by many others including

'N Sync. His follow up albums were just as good as his first, but he could not compete against multi-talented behemoths pitching sex and a six pack.

WHO SETS THE STANDARDS?

I am a father of a teenage year boy and I know what he is in for. Let me explain. Speaking to you teens in particular for a moment if I may. You are under the most aggressive attack of sex in the media that history has ever seen. You can hardly watch a commercial for chewing gum without seeing some ultra-sexy model in it. Magazines, television shows, nearly everything you see is an assault on your self-body consciousness. The media is basically telling you what's hot and what's not...and I fear for those of you who buy into such nonsense. For all of you who have struggled with food to the point of disorder for the sake of "image" let me say this; it is not worth it, period. If you are considering that as a course of action, I urge you to get help immediately and seek counselling.

COMPLACENCY

On the other extreme of image is the philosophy that you should just accept your body and be happy with what you look like, no matter what. I agree with a great deal of that philosophy, but I also disagree with some of it. Truth of the matter is that if you are not happy with something, even your body, you should change it, but not because anyone told you to do so. I know a lot of people who are considered to be (or think they are) "overweight" who are far healthier in both body and mind than many lean or "skinny" people. You alone should determine what your weight goals are and what you want to look like. No one should dictate that to you.

I would not say anything to you that I do not have first hand experience with. I was not happy at over 300 lb. and a size 56 waist. If I had decided to "accept my body" the way it was I'd probably be miserable right now, as well as possibly diabetic, or worse. Each of us is different in the way we think and what is important to us—that is a wonderful diversity we possess. However, if you are of the mind that you do want to lose fat and change your body for whatever reasons are important to **you,** then let me encourage you: You **can** do it! I want to gently and respectfully remind you about who is writing here. I am not a ripped-six-pack-cover-model-since-birth guy and I have fought a lot of the same battles you are facing and I have won. I am probably no smarter than you are. I just learned about food, about exercise, and I worked with a fitness professional for a while and I did it. If you possess the skills needed to read this book, then you also possess the skills to take control of your life and lose the fat.

If any of the fast-food chains sported an image of what a person might look like if they ate their food as much as they actually wanted you to, they would go out of business. If you have not seen the film *Super Size Me* then I whole-heartedly recommend that you do and you'll see what I mean!

SETTING REALISTIC EXPECTATIONS

When I did decide to start working out at a gym regularly, I enlisted the help of a trainer who was instrumental in educating me. The first thing he did was ask me to come in with pictures from magazines of what I hoped to look like. It was important for me to have an image in my head and to also help me set realistic expectations. I am an endomorph (that is a technical anatomical term for someone who can pack on muscle quickly, but can pack on fat just as fast). I came in with 12 pictures of my "dream physique," the first ten were of fashion models. He flipped through those ten rather quickly saying, "no, no, no, **definitely** no," until he came to pictures of guys who were bigger than those models, but had some muscle. When he saw those last two pictures, he looked up at me and smiled saying: "**this,** we can do." His insight was invaluable in helping set realistic goals, as well as what may have looked nice but was genetically impossible and flat out wrong for my body type. I am so thankful to Magnus for doing that; it saved me a lot of frustration. Bro, if you are reading this book, call me up! Would love to talk to you!

Back to "images" for a moment. Picture someone you think is really fit and a attractive to you chowing down on a 1200 calorie fat-filled hamburger, do you think it's "a hot guy/girl having a burger"? Picture an overweight person eating the same thing and it's: "wow, what a pig." We don't stop to think at how unhealthy the food is, we stop at how the person looks. This further illustrates my point that lean and skinny does not necessarily mean "fit" or "healthy."

SETTING UNREALISTIC EXPECTATIONS

I accompanied a friend of mine on a visit to his massage therapist and as I sat in the waiting room waiting, I picked up a copy of a popular magazine whose primary reading target was teenage girls. On the front cover was the caption "get a smoking hot bod in two weeks." I thought to myself: "**this,** I have **got** to see." So I turn the page, and there was a fitness model doing lunges, squats, and host of other exercises that were indeed, great ways to tone up a body. The problem is that if the reader that was going to be doing those same exercises wanted to lose say 15 lb., there was no way it was going to happen in two weeks. They made no mention in the article about good eating habits or expectations, but the "image" sure looked good. Publishing articles like that goes a long way to shattering already frail self-esteems in teens when they find out that the "two week hot bod" is nowhere to be found. As a result, they can feel like hopeless cases that will never lose weight.

PRODUCT ASSOCIATION

Commercials for razors are among my favourite for their use of images. This picture perfect guy with the Dick Tracy square jaw and washboard abs wakes up (with perfect hair of course) and picks up a razor. Lights flash, groovy music blares, all these words like "power," "sexy," etc. roll from script and then of course, the most stunning woman I have ever seen shows up behind the guy. Question: why does this not happen to me when I shave?

What if that was a "fat guy"? Don't fat guys shave too? I did! Would the razor not work properly? Is there no groovy music for him? What about the girl, is there at least a girl? Probably not. "IMAGE." Okay, I know it's a commercial to sell a product; I am just stressing my point further as to how "picture perfect" body images are thrown at us from every direction.

The only image you should be concerned with is the one YOU think is right for you. Don't let anybody sell you their ideal.

Fat Has Lousy Aim!

The effects of being overweight and morbidly obese are well documented these days. Any research compiled by a certified medical or fitness organization will provide you with reams of information about how being overweight will affect your immune systems and quality of life, and how the wrong food choices can set you up for Type 2 diabetes, as well as a host of other health complications.

FAT NEVER FORGETS

But fat is a poor shot. When it fires, the "bullets" hit a lot more than just our bodies, they wreak havoc on our minds as well.

In my case, I knew that being so overweight presented a risk to my health, but that was not my primary concern at the time. In fact, my chief concern was that I hated the way I looked and I barely gave the possible health risks any "weight" at all. (Pun intended!)

I hated myself. I would go out of my way to avoid being in pictures, and instead offered to take pictures of others. (Not a great compromise since I am a lousy photographer!) It all crippled me to the point of not wanting to go out of the house or on vacation. And, oh, forget about getting me within a country mile of a beach! When I did have the unfortunate and gruelling opportunity to have to see myself in a photo, I always noticed that I would cross one arm in front of my big fat gut and perhaps even pull my jacket around my size 56 waist enough to (hopefully) minimize the exposure.

Years later, after dropping 140 lb and keeping it off, I now look at myself in pictures and see **the very same thing.** No, that's not a typo, though I wish it were. Even now at a healthy weight, I still revert to the same tactics. Why? Since a lot of the time I still SEE that fat guy! The impact of being overweight hit my mind harder than it hit my body. I recovered and rescued my body, but the wounds to the ego and self-esteem were absolutely and by far the deepest and most devastating.

A bit of irony here, if I may...

Of all the people who could wind up falling in love with me, it had to be a National Fitness Champion.

"Are you KIDDING me?"

Enter Susan, a 36-year-old, all-natural dynamo who had two teenage kids via natural child birth and had a physique envied by every female (and a lot males) out there. She had (and still has) abs that you could grate a brick on.

Just my luck, huh?

When I met Susan, I had already been through the biggest period of my fat loss battle and had kept the weight off for several years. She pursued me vigorously, but I resisted. There were several reasons for my initial refusal of her advances and one of them was that I still "felt" fat. I was convinced that any time she would hug me and rub my chest or back that she was looking for muscle and was perhaps thinking to herself "this guy's body is all blubber." I was wrong, of course, but at the time, that was how I felt.

I can't even speak of what happened when I fell in deeply love with her and we became more intimate. Can you even imagine how I felt? You can read more about that later in the chapter "Susan, the Last Thing I Ever Expected."

A slew of people, from consultation clients, to friends and colleagues have said in one way or another, "You look incredible Marco, you don't even look like the same person!" Yet here I was/am, still fighting the fat monster. I could not bend over to tie my shoes for years and you know what? Now that I can, out of habit I still very rarely do. It just got "programmed" into the hard wiring of my brain.

WHO IS TO BLAME?

I still get all the isms. I get up and pull my shirt over my butt. Even as I hold fitness consultations in my office, I catch myself grabbing at my shirt to make sure it is not clinging to my stomach. I find myself reacting to my "memory of fat" several times in an hour. I actually call my client's attention to it and we have a laugh about it, but believe me, I don't do it on purpose.

Before I lost the weight, I was a pretty nice guy. I had a good heart and was honest…but I was fat. People make assumptions and in my case, they were right. I had to face the hard fact that I was out of control and that all the negative things people said about my body were, in fact, true.

Please get your head out of the sand, folks! Barring genetic issues or serious health complications, when people call us fat, as painful as it is to admit, they are right. If we are in a state of being overweight, or even morbidly obese, the fact is that we actively or (more likely) passively, *decided* to go there. We "invested" in a lifestyle, and in turn, our bodies yielded a return based on *exactly* what we put into them.

Whether it was abusing emotional eating to fight back at the way we may have *been* abused, or just flat out laziness, poor food choices or becoming couch potatoes, the stinging truth is that we have no one to blame but ourselves. Yes, we can blame our parents, but how long can we honestly do that for? When we reach the point of being able to think for ourselves and take action that reason just becomes an excuse, which finally becomes a crutch. Let me tell you—in my consultations, I have met people who have been leaning on and crushing that crutch (with all the weight of their fat), for a lifetime!

TOUGH CHANGES

At some point, we have to take ownership of our actions and decisions and finally make changes. No diet, no doctor, and not even this book can do it for you. Your success or failure is entirely in *your* hands.

What are you going to do this time around? Will this be the time when you take, perhaps, a baby step forward? Or are you going to landslide back to the bottom of the hill to whine and suffer some more?

Harsh words, I know. It took harsh moments to propel me to at least decide to change.

"The greatest risk is not taking one." I don't know who said that, but wow, is it ever true. If you are going to go down, then do so swinging with all your might. Don't just sit there and complain that it never worked for you without at least first trying. And try the *right* way! Don't complain and be miserable because some ridiculous starvation diet, magic pill, injection or "fat melting" lotion didn't work for you... none of these are *supposed* to work for you in the first place. The bottom line here (and it is unquestionably true) is: the only surefire way to start to lose weight is to eat sensibly, exercise regularly, and to do so for the rest of your life.

Get educated about healthy eating and exercise.

Then? *Do it! Period.*

You cannot be the only person on earth it doesn't work for, you are just not that special.

As for me, I am a little bit more comfortable in pictures these days, but I am still a horrible photographer!

My Friend Eats Anything She Wants and Never Gains Weight!

Let me introduce you to two friends, we'll call them Sue and Deb.

Sue and Deb are exactly the same age, within six months of each other. Sue is 5 ft. 2 and Deb is the same height. They both have two children each delivered via natural child birth. Both of them eat relatively healthy food and grew up within ten blocks of each other. There is one noticeable difference, however. Even with all of those similarities, Sue weighs 125 lb. while Deb weighs 200 lb.

Why is it that Deb that needs to "go on a diet," but not Sue?

METABOLISM

Okay, ladies, I have focused this chapter on you because I have heard more women than men say "if I even *look* at food, I gain weight." Since I firmly believe that women are not to be regarded merely as child-bearing and -rearing "machines" and also I happen to think that in a lot of areas, they are *way* smarter than us guys. I am going to explain metabolism to you ladies using what has been historically classed as a "guy" topic. Yup, that would be cars. Let me stop to say that most women and most men know more about cars than I do.

The "Sue Car" is a Ferrari, a car built for speed and performance. Its engine revs high and as a result, burns the energy (the fuel it stores) quickly.

The "Deb Car" on the other hand is more of a luxury car like a high end Buick. It is built for comfort and long trips and it stores energy (fuel) longer than "Ferrari Sue."

Let's call the piece of equipment that burns energy in these cars the motors.

Let's call the motor of your body the metabolism.

Sue and Deb have the same components, in theory, but the horse power, number of cylinders, and their performance levels are unique. They are both people, but the rate at which they consume their gas (energy) is different.

Let's bring it full circle here. Each of our bodies burns and/or stores energy differently, just as cars burn fuel differently. People with metabolisms (motors) that run at a faster rate, burn off excess fat and energy faster than those with slower motors. It is very important to understand this point. Once you have realized this, it is a quick and prudent leap to understanding that this is the very reason why one diet does not work for everyone. Please, read that again, it will set you free.

A word to the wise here; this does not mean that one person, by default, is necessarily any healthier (at least, internally) than the other. Overall health and/or well-being are not solely defined by maintaining a healthy weight. We must strive for wellness of mind and body as well as spirit. It is how each of our bodies handles the "gas" we feed it that determines the rate at which we store fat/energy, or burn it.

Imagine our Ferrari had a rotting motor in it. It would still *look* sexy, but is the car going to run with any amount of efficiency?

Whether you have a "Ferrari" or "Buick" type of metabolism, the good news is that both of these motors can run at peak efficiency, provided they are fed and maintained with high grade parts and "nutritious" fluids and components. This, in the case of our bodies, translates to healthy and nutritious foods and liquids.

Stored energy (by way of massive food intake) is what fuels the hibernation process of a bear. Bears have metabolisms that are comparatively faster than other animals that hibernate. As a result, bears have to eat *a lot* of food in order not to starve to death as they hibernate. Do you see the comparison here? Even though a bear is an omnivore who gains as much as 125 lb. in his preparation to hibernate, his metabolism (his motor) operates at such a high rate that, over the winter, he is in danger of starving. Why? Because a high metabolism burns "fuel" (energy) just like a performance car motor does.

CARBS! YES, OR NO?

We as humans, also eat food that provides energy largely in the form of *carbohydrates*. You may be more familiar with the term, "carbs." Low carb and no carb diets have been the on and off rage for over 30 years. It is not a new thing.

The concept behind a low-carb diet is quite simple. You eliminate food that can be kept in your body as stored energy and instead eat only proteins and fats (which burn off faster than carbs both due to the very composition of the food, as well the speed of your metabolism). The theory is that once most of the stored energy in your body has been removed, the body is then free to go after whatever fat is left. In essence, the body eats itself from the inside out. The dangers that are associated with this type of diet are well-documented and it is my opinion that you should absolutely not engage in such a diet unless your doctor prescribes you to do so for medical reasons. Even in that case, I would get a second opinion.

I did not write this book to debunk diets, but I *am* going to caution you to stay away from something that could potentially yield unfriendly and unforeseen results to your health in the long run. While the low carb idea does have some merit, the over-the-top amounts of bad cholesterol and fats you would eat on such a diet are alarming. Artery clogging fat and cholesterol is just not the way to go, folks. You might get leaner, but you will not get healthier. It is safe to say that not enough carbs or too many carbs are both extremes that should be avoided.

Remember: "everything in moderation."

Back to our "Car Gals." The good news is that it is, in fact, possible to rev your metabolism, causing it to burn stored energy and consume fat more efficiently. How do we hyper-charge our metabolism? We exercise, feed it high grade foods, and add lean muscle tissue.

There are different types of carbs and the great news (Susan says) is we can eat them all as part of a healthy eating plan.

Even with all the experience and knowledge I have amassed, at the moment I could not tell you how many calories to ingest. Such an assumption on my part, without having interviewed you and assessed you, would be completely irresponsible. The idea of prescribing the number of calories to consume to someone who hasn't been properly assessed raises a question or ten as to the legitimacy and effectiveness of telemarketed one size fits all" diets. Only a qualified and unbiased nutritionist (not one who works for a specific company that tries to sell you *their* food), can give you the right advice. That, in conjunction with an exercise plan (provided by a registered fitness professional) is what will enable you trade your "Buick" in for a "Ferrari."

Vroom vroom!

A Simple Plan

So, how do we start making these simple changes?
Here is part of my personal experience...

SMALL CHANGES, BIG RESULTS

I knew that eating an entire bag of chips was probably not a good idea. I was not ready to give up those chips, so I decided to start making some small changes by maybe eating half the bag. That for me was major progress and represented the very beginning of my success. You may think it ridiculous that I considered that eating only *half* a bag was *progress*, but to me it was.

After I got down to half a bag, I thought: do I need to eat this junk every day? Here's a thought—how about I have that half bag every *other* day instead? Again, it might seem ridiculous to call that progress. What you may not have considered is how that one simple move or baby step took over 4,000 calories of extremely high fat and bad cholesterol inducing agents out of my weekly way of eating. That was a staggering 16,000 calories less a month.

> Here's the math:
> 1 bag of chips (I am talking about the BIG bags) = 1,600 calories
> 5 bags per week = 8,000 calories
> So my weekly caloric intake of just those chips was 8,000 .
> I then decided to have *half* a bag of chips each day.
> I divided the 1,600 calories in half and was left with 800 calories.
> So I was then taking in half a bag (800 calories) 5 times a week.
> My weekly caloric intake became 4,000. That is already *half* of the 8,000 I was taking in earlier.
> Finally, I decide to eat that half bag every other day. Let's be generous and base this on a full week (7days). That means I'd be eating that half bag 3 times per week. Based on our earlier math of 800 calories per half bag, we can now multiply that by our 3 days.

Grand total: 2,400 calories per week. By the way, that's roughly the same amount of calories as in a single big combo type meal at your local fast food eatery!

To sum it up:
I began at 8,000 calories per week.
Then, by reducing to half a bag, I dropped to 4,000 calories per week and finally, by going to half a bag every other day, I slashed that to 2,400 per week.
Thinking exponentially, the monthly figures break down as follows:
I went from 32,000 calories monthly to 9,600. The grand total difference is a staggering 22,400 calories.
How is my baby step *progress* looking now? More like a *gigantic* leap!
Astounding, isn't it? Something so simple, such a small move yielded staggering results. Know what else? I lost some fat along the way and I had yet to do anything that even remotely resembled exercise.
I made a *small* change, I took a baby step and I lost fat.

TAKING IT FURTHER

Imagine now, that we also did one hour of medium to high intensity workout (weights and cardio). Let's be *really* generous and say we burned 1,500 calories (that is very high) in that workout. We can see that to burn those same 22,400 potato chip calories would take a *long* time. That is an extreme example, but it is a good concept to keep in mind.

CREATIVE LABELING

You can do this with just about anything that would be termed fast-food: sodas and soft drinks, etc. Here's how:
Next time you pick up a bottle of your favourite cola, flip it and have a look at the "nutrition facts" label. Now there are sneaky things to watch for here. If you are holding a 1 litre bottle of pop and the "total calories" on it are listed as 180, then you need to look at the label more closely. You will no doubt see the caption "per serving" and you will also be informed of what that product considers to be "one serving."
If the label reads: 180 calories per 100 ml (millilitre) serving and it is a 1 litre bottle of pop, then by downing the entire bottle you are not taking in 180 calories are you? Just what *are* you taking in then?
Some simple math to the rescue:

There are 1000 millilitres in one litre.

Your bottle contains that same amount.

The serving (or portion) size is based on 100 ml.

The label is telling us we are taking in 180 calories *each time* we consume just 100 ml of that cola. The information is staring you right in the face, but the company assumes you are too stupid or lazy to read, much less understand it!

If we take that serving size of 100 ml and multiply it by 10, we will have a grand total of 1000 ml (one litre)—that's our entire bottle.

So then this means it would take us 10 servings (according to the label's per serving information) to consume the entire bottle of pop.

So, 180 calories per serving x 10 servings = 1,800 calories, if the whole bottle is consumed.

Downing that entire bottle does not mean a total intake of 180 calories; it means a whopping 1,800 calories!

That means that if a particular individual's (remember, everyone burns calories differently, this is just an example) total caloric requirement for the day might be around 2,200 calories (to maintain current weight), then by downing that bottle of pop, that person has just taken in over 80% of that in calories that are going to go a long way to making him/her unfit and overweight.

There is no way a cola company is going to tell you on their label that you are about to ingest nearly 2,000 calories that are really bad for you. Remember, they just want to sell you their product, regardless of the consequences to your health or waistline.

THE CALORIES THAT SNEAK IN

These may seem to be extreme examples to some, but how many times have you ordered a large cola at a movie theatre and, without even knowing it, ingested about 48 tablespoons of sugar and over 1000 calories? That's not even making mention of the 1000 or so "bad" calories from the popcorn popped in palm kernel or coconut oil (humongous fat content in both, by the way). When you think of it that way, you might agree that my examples are in fact not extreme at all. If we look around us, all of these fat producing, artery clogging and cholesterol raising calories are as close as the nearest burger, Mexican food, or fried chicken drive-through.

I am not a math-whiz, not by a long shot. A simple calculator with the proper values inserted can help you realize what you are *truly* eating. Remember, check the "per serving" information on the nutrition label of the products you pick up as you shop. Go to your fridge or cupboard, pull out a packaged item, and try the calculation yourself. More often than not, you will be stunned by what you discover. You will find many of the "phantom" calories that are guilty of making sure you not only maintain your weight but also increase it via the calories you didn't even know you were eating.

SMALL REDUCTIONS

Another small change I began to make was in the way I took my coffee. I used to take my coffee double cream and double sugar. (In Canada it is commonly referred to as "double double.") As in my previous example of the chips, I decided to start slowly cutting back on the sugar in my coffee. I did not eliminate the sugar entirely, but instead of two teaspoons, I tried 1¾ tsp. Know what? It still tasted like the two teaspoons I was used to, but I wound up taking some more of those "phantom" calories out of my daily eating. I did the same thing with the cream and found I could handle the reduction just fine. Not everyone will wind up doing what I did, but the following example goes a long way to showing that we are all capable of doing things we never thought imaginable, just by trying. Just like every inch gained on a football field can add up to scoring a touchdown, the small food and lifestyle choices we make will ultimately make a big difference...good or bad!

Currently, I take my coffee with no sugar and I alternate between just black, skim milk, or cream the odd time. As a matter of fact, if sugar does wind up in my coffee I can't really drink it since the taste of the sugar now actually bothers my palate. Seems crazy, but it's true. I just tried something different from what I was accustomed to and found out that in the long run I liked it more than the way I was used to. Yes, folks, you can recondition your taste buds.

Some basic knowledge can put you in control of your weight, just give it a try. Start small and do not set goals that are overwhelming; drastic changes send your body into shock and withdrawals and will almost certainly guarantee failure.

Easy Does It

Once we are properly informed about nutrition and exercise and we put that education to use, weight loss is no longer some elusive thing that few can achieve—rather, it becomes easy.

That is not to say that shopping for healthy foods will instantaneously be easy or that picking the right food in a "spur of the moment" eating situation will come naturally. We are not wired to make these choices instinctively. It is a discipline, a way of life, that must first be learned and then consistently honed.

I want to remind you at this point that I do not hold any degrees in nutrition and yet, I was able to not only lose the weight, but keep it off, all by learning about what was going into my mouth and how to exercise. You can do so as well, make no mistake about that.

"Easy does it" is the approach we should take when moving from an unhealthy, overweight lifestyle to an active lifestyle where we are looking and feeling the way we always wanted to.

WALK BEFORE YOU CAN RUN

Those of us who follow tennis are routinely awed by the serving power of Andy Roddick. This guy can blast howitzer missile serves at an opponent at a staggering 155 mph. As a former tennis player myself, I know that such a talent can be devastating to even the most skilled opponent.

Let's assume for the moment that I indeed had the *potential* to strike a ball at such speeds. Is that where I start? (I wish.) No, I start by learning how to hold a racket and hit the ball and then hopefully make progress in both power and accuracy.

Let's apply the same principle here. When I was really overweight, I used to see guys on magazine covers with ripped abs and toned physiques. Similarly, all of the ladies on magazine covers were stunning and had perfect legs, waistlines, and butts. I used to think two things: "I'd love to look even *half* as good as that guy. Man, if I could lose even just a measly 10 lb., I'd feel so much better about myself." My second thought was that I'd never have the six pack of abs; it was just not possible for me. As I sit here and write to you, my dear reader, I still do not have that ripped six pack, but it has begun to form.

Let's be honest here, the people you see on these magazine covers are models. Their mission in life is to look as good as possible so they can be hired for cover shoots and subsequently sell magazines. Now I gotta ask, is that what *you* do for a living? Do you have endless hours to put in at the gym and to watch everything that goes into your mouth? Some top notch models/actors even have nutritionists and chefs working for them, or have healthy meals that fit into their eating plan pre-made and delivered to them.

Do you have that kind of lifestyle and are your pockets that deep? That is simply not reality for most of us.

Having said that, I knew I wanted and needed to lose fat. So I had a choice...I could sign up at a gym and take a stab at it (clueless as I was) and then go on a regimented eating plan to achieve that six pack of abs, or I could look at the reality of my lifestyle and start taking some simple steps.

I decided to first "pick up the racket and learn to simply hit the ball." Baby steps..."easy does it."

Step out onto a tennis court and try to pound a serve at even 100 mph without ever having picked up a racket and observe what will happen to you. Lots of pain, lots of potential for injury, and an acute sense of failure followed by feeling like "this is impossible. I'll never even get the ball over the net!" (You will also more than likely look *very* silly. But hey, just wear nice clothes; fashion goes a long way!)

POINT YOURSELF IN THE RIGHT DIRECTION

Oh sure, my long-term goal was to lose over 100 lb. but I wasn't even moving in that general direction. In fact, I wasn't *moving* at all.

In the simplest of examples, let's assume I want to go to Florida from Toronto, Canada. The direction to travel to get there is decidedly south. Therefore, what is my very first move? *Turn* to face south! It is the simplest of moves, yet it is vital! No use in facing north, east, or west now, is there?

Want to get healthier? Face the direction of the road that will get you there! Point yourself and make the simplest of moves to travel in that general direction. Primarily—move! Walk! Take the stairs once in a while. What? You say it's tough? Well consider this: the very first day I stepped on a treadmill I went for three minutes and rapidly proceeded to toss my cookies. I threw up violently! Discouraged? Absolutely! Undaunted, the next day I went back and tried it again. Know what happened? Exactly the same thing! Yup, three minutes and I was off to ride the "porcelain train." Discouraged? EVEN MORE than the previous day! I went back for a third go and this time I made it to three minutes. "Baby Steps!" On day four, I added five seconds to that time. I aimed to add one minute per week. *I didn't always make it, but I didn't give up, either.* Today I can blast through an hour of intense cardio and leave people half my age sampling a taste of the bottoms of my running shoes. Did I *start* there? Did Andy Roddick *start* by blasting tennis balls so fast they are nearly invisible? Nope! Andy and I started in much the same fashion. (Bro, if you ever read this, I think you are awesome!)

Just get moving. Start small. Even small is better than nothing at all!

Food or Faux?

Before we begin, it is important to understand our subject matter. In this chapter, we will be dealing with food.

FOOD a definition:
Material, usually of plant or animal origin that contains essential nutrients such as carbohydrates, fats, proteins, vitamins, or minerals and is ingested and assimilated by an organism to produce energy, stimulate growth, and maintain life.

Source: The American Heritage® Stedman's Medical Dictionary Copyright © 2002, 2001, 1995 by Houghton Mifflin Company. Published by Houghton Mifflin Company.

In looking at the above definition a little more closely, we can see words such as "essential nutrients" followed by carbohydrates, fats, proteins, etc. These three make up what has generally become known as the three food groups. Reading a little further we see the words "to produce energy, stimulate growth, and maintain life." In all of my exhaustive research, I have yet to come across a definition of food that includes terms such as "to help you lose weight" or "to help you gain weight." Indeed, that is not food's primary function and so called "health" or "diet foods" do not exist. There is conclusive proof, however, that what we eat and how much of it we eat has a direct effect on our fitness, energy, well-being, and yes...weight.

IS IT FOOD, OR JUST SOMETHING WE EAT?

What is of major concern is just how the very word "food" has been changed and "packaged." If we were to believe all the ads in print, on television, and on the Internet, we would have to be of the mind that everything being pitched to us is in fact, "food." But, is it *really* food? Or is it more just *something we eat*? Do the ingredients of some of the "food" in these ads in any way resemble the purpose of food as we saw in our previous definition? Are the foods in these ads "essential nutrients…ingested… to produce energy, stimulate growth, and maintain life"?

Now, let me stop here for a moment to remind you that I was born in Italy, and that we are lovers of food. So, although tiramisu (a rich coffee cheesecake-type dessert) serves very little purpose as a "nutrient," the taste can soon make you forget about that. Let's just remember what we discussed earlier: "everything in moderation."

THE ASSAULT

So let's come back to our current discussion by way of example.

It's 8:00 p.m. and there you are in your La-Z-Boy chair watching television. You are not even thinking about food at the moment, as you had dinner not more than two hours ago. Your program breaks for commercials and, WHAMMO, there it is! We are talking about the assault on your wallet, the assault on your senses, and the battle for control of your child's diet (through toys given away freely with a meal). Commercial follows commercial beaming images of chips, beer, fast food burgers and fries, ice cream…and, amazingly enough, none of the people in the ads look to be an ounce overweight and most of them are gorgeous. Amazing, isn't it? Sign me up!

CATCH PHRASES

Let's have a look at some of the "catch phrases" which are all so familiar to us by now.

"Contains no added MSG" - Fine, so there's no *added* MSG. That does not mean there isn't enough naturally occurring MSG already in the product to drop a horse.

"Made from real fruit juice" - Oh, so it is not *real* fruit juice…but it is *made from* real fruit juice. Why not just sell me real fruit juice! Just what the heck are they putting in there if it's not 100% real fruit?

"Low in fat" - Does that mean that it's also low in cholesterol? How about refined sugars and calories? What else is in there other than this "low fat"? How about the fact that we actually *need* certain fats in our everyday diet?

"Part of a balanced breakfast" - "Balanced" you say? Balanced according to whom? According to companies who stand to profit from the sale of this "food." Do they bother to mention the amount of tooth rotting sugar in this "balanced" breakfast?

Whether or not you read the Bible, there is a scripture in it that is one of the most accurate statements ever made. It reads: "people perish for lack of knowledge." In the colloquial, we can read this as; people get burned because they are ignorant and uninformed. I am hard-pressed to think of a more appropriate area to cite this scripture than in the area of food and nutrition.

Unless you are a mechanic or good with cars, think of what happens when you need to get your car serviced. Do you lack the knowledge to fix it yourself? If so, your ignorance puts you at the mercy of a mechanic. Hopefully you work with an honest one. The same goes for trusting a food product advertisement. If you are uneducated, you are at the mercy of what they are telling you.

Do we just believe what advertisers are telling us? Did they go out and do all of the research so they could sell us food that is good for us? Or could it be possible that they are in this to make money, regardless of the benefit or harm to us? The TV stations, print media, and Internet carry the ads for these companies for that same reason—profit.

We are either going to educate ourselves or just blindly believe that what these food and advertising companies are telling us is the truth. Will you believe that they are also making the best nutrition choices possible on our behalf?

Based on what you have just read, are you willing to take that chance?

Make the distinction. Is it "food" or just something to eat?

Calorie Confusion

You've heard it all before: watch your calories, count your calories, low calorie, high calorie, reduce your calories. What *is* a calorie then? I am glad you asked!

Now since I set out to write a book that would be simple to read and understand, I am not going to launch into a study on how calories and nutrients are produced through photosynthesis of the sun interacting with plants etc. Here then is the most basic explanation I can offer.

First of all, calories are marvelous things and they are good things. Without calories, we would cease to exist. Keep that in mind the next time you consider going on a low-calorie or starvation diet.

WHERE DO ALL THOSE CALORIES GO?

Think of calories as little pockets of energy that fuel your body. Your body needs a minimum amount of calories in order for it to function, similar to the way a car requires energy through gas and oil in order to run efficiently. As humans, we obtain this energy through food, which contains "calories" a unit of energy.

Once again using a car engine for sake of comparison, a motor uses up or "burns" the energy in the fuel it is "fed" in order to function and move. Similarly, our bodies "burn" calories to do the same thing. The calories or energy is burned by way of our metabolism (see the "My Friend Eats Anything She Wants" chapter). "Metabolism" is the "motor" inside our bodies. **Just as each car motor burns or uses energy differently, each of our bodies also burn calories in a way that is unique to our metabolism.**

When we eat food, calories go through a chemical process in our bodies until they are either absorbed for immediate use, or conserved in our bodies as stored or saved energy. Some stored energy is required for everyday survival, but too much of it just sits there, doing nothing and turning to fat. If a car is parked at the end of the day and there is still gas (energy) in its tank, what is the point of that? The gas is just sitting there, stored and doing nothing. Basically, it's in reserve.

Each of us requires a minimum number of calories in our bodies in order to breathe, think, and, in essence, sustain life. The minimum number of calories each of us requires to maintain or lose weight is unique to each individual, though there are some averages. Let's assume you are an individual who requires 2,000 calories each day in order for your body to maintain its ideal weight and perform the other tasks needed throughout the day. What happens if you take in more or fewer calories than your body burns? Quite simply, you will either gain or lose fat (stored energy) respectively. So by way of simple math:

CALORIC CONVERSION

If your body needs to burn 2,000 calories each day to survive and you take in 2,500, you then have an excess of 500 calories that are just sitting there waiting to be used up. If you do that long enough and store enough of those calories, they will wind up as pounds of fat and will usually make their home right around your face, belly, butt, and the backs of your arms more than anywhere else.

On the other hand if you choose to exercise, at least some of the stored energy you have will be called on by your body and burned instead of sitting in reserve. When you exercise and use up those "stored deposits" of fat and energy, you lose weight. This is not a theory, it is a fact.

The more "stored energy" you have that is just sitting there in reserve, the more weight your body will keep and carry. Imagine now that you take in 500 calories more than your body can burn daily for a month (not a hard thing to do by way of junk food). What you will be left with is 15,000 extra units of unused energy (calories) in your body. This is the process that a bear uses in order to survive hibernation throughout the winter. Bears pack on as much as 150 lb. doing this. Get the picture? The BIG, FAT picture?

There is a school of thought that is generally accepted which states that 3,500 calories are needed to create 1 lb. of fat. For our purposes here, let's suppose this is true. Using our bear example above, 15,000 unused calories in a month represents a weight gain of just less than 4 1/2 lb. Do that for a year and you are talking about roughly 50 lb. total in unhealthy weight gain. How would you look and feel if you *lost* 50 lb.? I'll bet a lot better than you do now.

REV YOUR METABOLISM

The amazing thing about exercise is that it revs your metabolism (fuel efficiency) and not only burns off more of the stored energy, but it leaves your motor running at an accelerated state, hours after you are done walking, lifting weights, whatever activity you took part in. Now then, you remember in Chapter 5, Sue Ferrari and Deb Buick? By exercising, even just walking briskly for 20 minutes, Deb has begun the "custom work" that will make her Buick metabolism burn fuel faster and leave less fuel in reserve. Deb is slowly moving towards "performance."

That is the good news here, you *can* get your metabolism to burn that fuel (stored energy) faster and with greater efficiency than it ever did before by "tuning it up" through "regular maintenance," which for our purposes we will call exercise and nutrition.

The bottom line here is that we have to "burn" more calories than we are storing and in doing so, weight loss *will* occur. That is a scientific fact.

Although this is indeed a fact, your body's ability to store and process calories will definitely be affected if you force your metabolism into a perceived state of starvation. Frequent meals are a key component in ensuring that your body will in fact "burn up" those extra stored calories. For more on this, please refer to chapter in this book entitled "Starving to be Fat."

Live and Let Die

We walk the supermarket aisles and there they are: the same "foods" on the shelves week after week. They look the same; they even taste the same...the only thing that will probably change is pricing and packaging. I live in Canada and yet I can travel across the ocean to Europe, walk the supermarket aisles there, and "presto" find the exact same cookie I can buy in Canada. What's more, I can come back to that same aisle months later and that same package may still be there. Amazing! Man has made things "better"; they have engineered a way to make "food" last longer!

My question to you then would be—is it *supposed* to last longer?

LOOKS CAN BE DECEIVING

Let's hold that thought for a moment as we consider the following.

Imagine you have gone shopping for groceries at your favourite store. You are walking up and down the aisles. What do you see? On the shelves there are boxes, shrink wrapped items, items in flashy eye-catching wrappings. Does any of that even *remotely* evoke thoughts of fresh, nutritious, or wholesome? Why are these items contained and wrapped in such a fashion? Two words: *preservation* and *profit.*

Now, let's take a walk through the "smaller" aisles. You know, the "quiet" aisles where there are no children begging, "Mom, can I get that?" Do you know where we are? Yes, we have entered the vegetables and fruits section! *(Go ahead and cue the Twilight Zone theme here for effect.)*

In this section of our supermarket, we see fruits and vegetables. We do not, however, see the flashy packaging we spoke of earlier, (actually, we see nature's own natural and flashy packaging). We do see all kinds of natural and vibrant colours along with varying sizes and textures. You think to yourself: "There doesn't seem to be 'selective placement' in this section like back in aisle six where all of the cereals loaded with sugars that include toy prizes were placed at eye level for three- to five-year-olds to see."

Come to think of it, there's no "sexy" packaging in this veggie and fruit section. How are they *preserving* all of this stuff?

Okay, trip is over, come on back here, get yourself some fruit and let's get back to our book.

Well, here's the deal: **Real, wholesome food is supposed to live and die.**

Yes, it **is supposed** to die, after which more food will grow and then also die **and so on**.... Man, however, has decided to put food on life support. Actually, **man decided** to create entirely new "food" that never even existed on **the earth up until** the last two centuries.

Call it God, **call** it Mother Nature, the fact is that an ingenious self-producing and reproductive food chain has existed since long before pre-packaged fast foods and preservatives. All we needed to do was tend to it and we would have been just fine and a LOT healthier than we all are right now. Well, how did we survive before the local supermarket? We survived on what I like to call "God's Natural Food Chain."

Sun, earth, and water did it all. The system was autonomous and it is still around today. Yet, by the 1950's we were in the middle of what the American Heart Federation called "an epidemic of coronary disease." What changed? In short: **everything!**

FOOD ON LIFE SUPPORT

A man started a restaurant and had an idea. His line of thought may have been something like, "If my burgers are selling this well in one city, imagine if I could sell this same type of burger in a bunch of other cities. Wow, the money I could make doing this would be amazing! Problem is that I don't have a factory to manufacture my product in each city, since that would be too expensive. So here's an idea: why don't I transport the food to other cities by truck or plane? If I can't get the food there quickly enough, it will go bad and rot. Thank God for preservatives!"

Know what, dear reader? Boy, did his idea ever work!

Preservatives and artificial ingredients can be found in all of our processed foods these days. Government food regulators have sanctioned the use of over 6,000 artificial agents for use in food processing, some of which either are, or contain, cancer inducing agents.

Let's have a look at classic. Cola, soft drink, whatever you have heard it called, it's basically chemical soup. Yet, watch how those crafty calories can sneak up on you via "friendly" food labeling.

SERVING SIZE

When you buy a can of cola, it's a safe bet to assume that you are planning to drink the entire contents of the can in a reasonably short period of time. Then please explain to me, why it is that the manufacturing company has provided you with nutrition information that is based on sips? Quite simply, if they actually placed a nutrition label clearly stating something along the lines of "if you drink this entire can, you will take in 450 calories and mostly all from sugar," how many cans of soda do you think they would actually sell?

Pretty clever strategy, isn't it?

"Oh, but it's *diet* soda", you say.

Well it may be "diet," but just what the heck *is* it? Can you read the first six ingredients on the can or bottle? Can you even *pronounce* the words? Do these ingredients even *look* like they are edible to you? When something is made in what is essentially **a chemical plant that hides behind a food brand name,** is what they produce something that you want to be putting into your body? Or your child's?

One of my mantras;

"If I can't read it, I won't eat it."

Go to the store and pick out some "low fat" cookies and have a look at the ingredients listed on the packaging. Do all of the ingredients look natural, or is the label rife with chemicals, acids, "golden" syrups, HFCS (High Fructose Corn Syrup), hydrogenated this or that oils, shortening, etc.?"

At some point, common sense must come into play when making choices as to what we are going to put into our bodies. It's all there in the ingredient labels. All of the information you need to make a wise or unwise choice is staring your right in the face. What are you going to do about it? Are you going to pick up a questionable item and feed it to yourself or your child, all for the sake of convenience? "Convenience," let's have a look at that concept.

IS FAST FOOD REALLY MORE CONVENIENT?

What takes longer to eat: an apple or a bag of potato chips? Which one is healthier for you to consume? (Hint: Pick the apple!). We could have all natural oatmeal in the morning (takes 90 seconds to heat), add a dash of real maple syrup and some fruits, instead of having boxed cereal and milk from a carton. You could make an incredibly delicious sandwich with veggies and perhaps some tuna, as opposed to a trans fat loaded, prepackaged, frozen hamburger, right? We can form good habits or bad habits.

Did you come from a box? Did you come frozen? Of course not! You came into the world as a living, breathing human being. Shouldn't you eat food that is natural, as opposed to it coming from a box or being frozen for months, if not years?

PERFECTION DID NOT NEED OUR HELP

Why does natural food have seeds? Why does it grow from the ground or on trees? It's pretty obvious that these elements are in place so that there could be a continuous supply of food, isn't it? Do cookies have seeds? What about chips and pop—do they? Well, of course not! The reason is that they never existed in nature until we created them.

Natural food arrived on our planet in a perfect state and it needed no help from us other than water and the planet took care of the sunlight and climates to help it grow. I hear all the environmentalists out there shouting and you are right; we are destroying the planet and in turn sabotaging our very own perfect food system. Even still, we have a far better chance of making healthier food choices if we go back to the food sources provided by the planet. We can either eat the real food or eat boxes and cartons containing lard and chemicals instead.

"Oh Marco, you are way too extreme. That's ridiculous!"

Well, considering I successfully navigated myself through a 140 lb. fat loss, you tell me: how extreme am I? Did my changes, my "extremities" yield results? Well, you are reading this book to find out how I did it, aren't you? I guess they must have worked after all!

If we go back to one of the oldest books in existence, the Bible, we can see many examples of all types of foods.

> *8 It is a land of wheat and barley, of grapevines, fig trees, pomegranates, olives, and honey.*
> *9 It is a land where food is plentiful and nothing is lacking.*
> *10 When you have eaten your fill, thank the LORD your God for the good land he has given you.*
> Deuteronomy 8:8–10. From *New King James Version*

Well, that's a whole lotta carbs now, isn't it!

Whether you believe in God, the planet, Vishnu, Mother Nature, or the Big Bang is not the question here. The point is that *real* food has been in place since man has existed and no religion, existential, or atheist belief can disprove that.

Choose *real* food, not something man created. Your body will thank you and take care of you.

Failing to Plan

Most of us have at least a general plan for the day ahead of us. Though we may not know the specifics of what lies ahead, we might know that we'll be at the mall by 1:00 p.m. or at the grocery store, dentist's office, etc.

One of the key factors that contributed to my weight gain in the past was a failure to plan my meals. I would plan my day out, knowing I'd be at such a location at a certain time, I'd probably need to wear this or that, I'd need to arrange for someone to watch my son while I was out, etc. One thing I never planned ahead was eating. It was never on a predetermined agenda and I have found this to be the case with nearly everyone I have spoken with about their weight gain experience.

Why is that? Why do we fail to even give food a second thought while planning out our day? Usually what winds up happening is something like this:

WHO WILL DECIDE WHAT YOU WILL PUT INTO YOUR BODY?

2:00 p.m. hits and you're thinking to yourself, I am *starving*! You look at your friend and say, "Wanna grab something?"

First of all, you may have not eaten since 8:00 a.m. (no wonder you are ravenous) and now you have put yourself in the perfect position to sabotage nearly any chance of eating healthy. By doing this you have taken the decision of controlling what you are going to eat completely out of your hands. You *have*, however, handed that decision over to the junk food places that surround you as you stand in the mall's food court. You are now completely at the mercy of their meal suggestions and their ideas, as well as your desperate and voracious appetite.

So what do you do? Chances are that you will order a salad of some type. Trouble is that salad may be carrying some 900 calories (which is nothing to say of the sulphites and other nasty preservative chemicals found in there).

Of all the things we plan, why do we not give any thought to food opportunities (or lack thereof) during the day? Well, here's some food for thought. Do we not think it is important enough an issue? We take time to plan and prioritize everything else it seems, except the one thing that directly affects our health, energy, and the stamina to even get *through* the day we have planned.

SIMPLIFIED FOOD PLANNING

Thinking ahead can go a long way to minimize the chances of sabotaging an otherwise healthy food plan. Here is an example of how I slowly integrated food planning into my life.

It's Monday night and I already know I am going to be on the road for most of the day tomorrow. Hey, I've got an idea, why don't I make an extra portion of whatever I am eating tonight to take with me tomorrow? Make an extra tuna sandwich tonight and pop it in a Ziploc bag and stick it in the fridge. Tomorrow, when I head out for my day I'll just take it with me. Sounds simple enough, right?

By making even this slight change, I kept myself in control of at least one food opportunity in the coming day. Tomorrow when I get hungry, I can take five minutes and have my sandwich. I know it is healthy and there is no chance that I will make an otherwise poor food choice. Doing so will also save me some money (not a bad thing).

Preparing an extra portion took very little time and is such a simple solution, yet I had never really stopped to do it before.

If we can reduce the opportunities of making poor food choices by minimizing the chance of even *finding* ourselves in compromising situations where we are not in control, we can radically enhance our chance for overall health and weight loss.

Make an effort to plan ahead. Can you imagine the kind of money (and calories) you will save by not eating out so often? Maybe you could start even entertaining "food planning" as a regular part of your life.

This did not come naturally for me; I really had to work at it. It felt a lot more natural to pull up to a drive-through and drop $10 on something totally unhealthy. Seemingly small steps at first will yield big results in the long run.

Decisions, Decisions

The most important piece of equipment that we have to lose weight and live healthy is not found anywhere in our muscles, but rather in the "muscle" between our ears. That is where the battle of weight loss and health is fought and won…or lost. Once we make a decision to do something about our fitness, we then need to act on our decision. "Faith without works is dead!" Amen! Trust me when I say that your muscles won't just pick up and start exercising all on their own, you must first decide and then act by making the physical effort of "moving."

The same goes for making healthier choices in the way we eat. Food does not just propel itself into our mouths all on its own, *we* put it there. If we overeat and lose sight of portion control, then praying to the heavens to "cast out" the calories, like they were some evil spirit, just won't work either. No mind trick in the world will change our way of eating, but there is no doubt that we can. By deciding to *eat sensibly for life*, we automatically remove the option of "falling off" of a diet, since we are not *on* one to begin with. This is a key and vital component to lifelong success.

YOU MUST TAKE CONTROL

In trying to define what eating sensibly for life is, ponder this thought:

If you go on vacation somewhere and are afraid you will gain weight, then you have not yet gotten a hold of portion control, and you have probably also not adequately educated yourself on the subject of food.

On one of our vacations, Susan and I wound up in the Dominican Republic at a five-star resort. The food was incredibly delicious and there was an over abundance of it. The decadent desserts were present, and they too, were also delicious and "irresistible." Okay, the last word in that sentence bugs me. Truth is, they are indeed "resistible," *if* you *choose* to exercise some restraint and discipline! Notice the emphasis on the words "if" and "choose," folks.

I think Susan and I actually came home leaner from that vacation. We did this by balancing our overall eating while still managing to indulge here

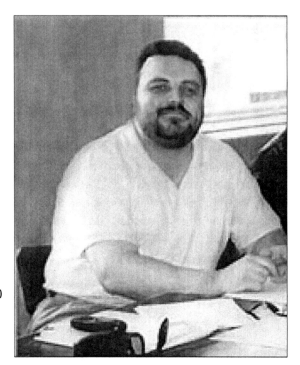

In New York, 1999. At this point, I had already lost close to 40 Lb. Wearing a size 54 pant , and hiding behind the table.

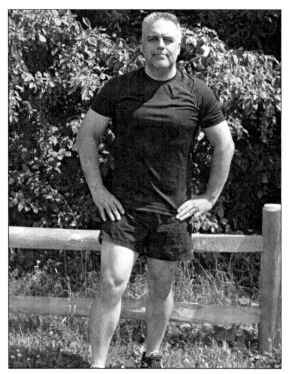

Ten years later, with size 36 pants, now too loose. How weight training changed my body.

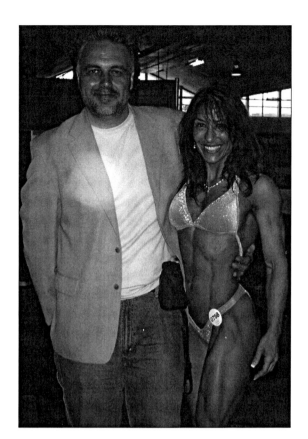

Marco and Susan at the FAME WORLD Championships, Toronto, 2007. Susan took 1st place in the figure category.

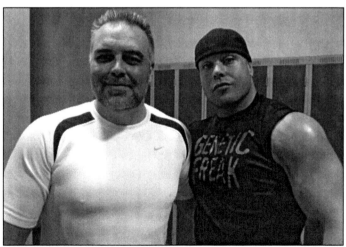

The reason for my pain, as well as a lot of my progress! Taken right after an intense training session with my trainer, Rob Thomson aka "The Test Express". June 2009.

and there.

Here's an example of one situation I found myself in where I could have gone with the flow, or decided to make some healthier food choices.

Some time ago, I ran into some old acquaintances and we decided to catch up over dinner. We wound up at a steak house and before long the menus arrived. The appetizer that my friends wanted to order fed four, but was made up entirely of deep fried onion. We are talking a cholesterol bomb here. There were other way healthier choices, so there I sat deciding until I settled on a plate of veggies with some cheese and spicy salsa. This may seem like such a simple example, but it is in situations such as the one I was in when you decide to take control of your health. In that situation, I had to make a decision about whether or not to tack an additional 700–1,000 calories (of the worst kind) onto my day. I had the same amount of time as my friends to survey the menu, the same choices to consider, and I *decided* to look after my health first. Regular and healthier choices made on a daily basis in situations such as this one can truly make it or break it.

Why did I opt out of the cholesterol bomb appetizer? Was it because the "diet" I was on didn't allow for it? Was it because I had used up all my "food points" for the day? (Some diets assign point values to food and give you a maximum of points to not exceed daily.) Actually it was neither reason. I opted out because I knew better. I had taken the time to educate myself about what was good for me to eat and what was bad.

REMEMBER WHO IS IN CONTROL

Sometimes we need to just remember the basics. No advertisement, food manufacturer, food packager, friend or restaurant has the power to force us to eat something. Having said that, how many times in the past have we empowered otherwise powerless agents to decide what we eat?

Can a car ad force you to buy a certain vehicle? No, they can only suggest that you do. Can a man or woman force another married individual into an extramarital affair? No, but the suggestion is there. Then why do the words: "I couldn't help myself, I lost control" find their way into our vocabulary? The truth of the matter is that we didn't just magically lose control, we *decided* to *give up* control and yield to whatever was beckoning us. Any circumstance is powerless. It is how we react and what we decide to do in any given situation that will determine how that circumstance will affect us.

Think of it this way: someone puts a loaded gun on a table, it's just sitting there. You can either pick it up and shoot somebody with it (please don't), or you can take the bullets out of it and put it away. The gun or circumstance has no power in and of itself, it's just "there." It is your reaction and decision that decides just what role that gun will take on.

THE BATTLE FOR YOUR DOLLARS AND SENSE

Food manufacturers spend a lot of money on research, demographics, etc. When this research is given a voice through advertising, their goal is to make your food choice for you. They decide to program your kids to want sugar-loaded cereal. Make no mistake, these companies are fully aware that what they want your kids to eat is not good for them. To ensure that your child tells mom or dad that they want a particular brand of "food," they will target and entice your child directly. How do they do this?

- They will draw up a cartoon character that is fun and colourful and tie it to a brand name.
- They will solicit merchandisers of major films, so as to include the likeness of characters from the movie on the cereal box.
- They will include toys and prizes in the cereal box itself.
- They will include phrases such as "reduced sugar" to make mom and dad feel better about the purchase. Truth is, even if half the sugar were removed from some cereals, there would still be enough of it to exceed what any child should consume (as a healthy amount).
- They will vie for high traffic "shelf placement" in grocery stores. They will make sure that their product will be on a shelf that is at eye- and reach-level for most kids aged 3–12.
- They will hire someone famous and "cool" to advertise their product.

Look at those points above; can any of those be considered a fluke? Not by any stretch of the word. These people want your kids' business now and in the future. These makers of junk food really do not care about the impacts on your child's health, but they *do* care about how much money they will make. Profit is the only direct goal of every business that exists, including food companies.

I am a single father of a boy in his teens, and, as such, the responsibility of shopping and cooking for him falls on me. One of the biggest changes I made with my boy was moving him from enriched (see definition in Chapter 19) white bread to whole grain bread. Why was there this resistance? Well, in part, it is because he was always fed white enriched bread at home in the past. No doubt that had a major impact. The rest of the matter is thanks to "food" advertising. When have you ever seen a peanut butter and jelly or bologna (that would be baloney) commercial where the featured bread is not white? I bet you can't think of one.

YOU DO, HOWEVER, HAVE A CHOICE.

We (along with our children) have been fed a suggestion and have been conditioned to eat enriched white bread. Who *decided* to *decide* for us? Was it the World Health Organization? No. Was it the United States Food and Drug Administration? No. Was it any health promoting corporation or agency? No. It was the food companies.

Make the decision that you are going to choose what you and your kids eat.

TALKING TO YOUR KIDS ABOUT HEALTHY EATING CHOICES

My son is a huge fan of the Star Wars movies (so am I). One of the ways I explained about the healthier choices we were making in our eating was to reverse the marketing ploys of some of the types of ads we discussed earlier in this chapter. I told my son the truth. Those amazing "Jedi Knights" or other superheroes or sports superstars did not get to be the way they are by eating enriched or processed foods. They got to be the way they are by eating *healthy* food and exercising. Once a child or a teen realizes this, they may very well try to emulate those healthy eating habits, along with all the other things they try to copy when it comes to their heroes. That's just a tactic that worked in my son's case.

The sexpot, rock hard bodies in rap and pop music did not come to be by eating junk food and not exercising. Yet, who do the hottest half-naked pop stars get endorsement deals from? Junk food companies, especially ones that manufacture calorie-laden sugar pop and sodas. Does anyone detect the *slightest* hint of hypocrisy here?

I say it again here: we need to get educated and understand just what we are eating. *We* need to make our own decisions. It is the only way.

People perish for lack of knowledge!

Horror Stories and Misconceptions, from my Life as a Fitness Consultant.

I always open my consultations with the phrase "this is the last job on earth I ever expected to have."

A guy that used to weigh over 340 lb. had a size 56 waist and 49 percent body fat, becomes a top fitness consultant for a major fitness company. I re-read that prior sentence and am still stunned—I still can't quite believe it!

In my position as a fitness consultant, I have spoken with thousands of people. As different as each of these precious people are, they nearly all have some common denominators. Here are a few of those common denominators, although the names of the actual people have been changed to maintain confidentiality.

LOSING FAT VS TONING UP

"Martha" came into my office weighing 485 lb. She was a sweet lady of 35 years and was desperate to lose weight, obviously. She had spent thousands of dollars at clinics and nothing had worked, so she had come to me looking for answers and I was able to give her some.

Of her total weight (485 lb.) her body fat percentage was a staggering 65 percent. This meant that she was carrying over 300 lb. of pure fat. Oddly enough, her approach was going to be the same as another person I had consulted who wanted to "tone up" and maybe lose only ten lb. Think it would work? Of course not. Funny thing is, the person wanting to tone up and lose just ten lb. also had the wrong approach. Both of these people decided they would just do cardio on a treadmill to lose weight. Truth is, they would indeed lose weight, but just *what* would they lose? Muscle or fat?

Muscle has three times the density of fat. A pound of lean muscle tissue can burn up to 50 calories per day while fat burns nothing, it just hangs and flaps there. In order to burn fat, lean muscle tissue *must* be present! Moving, aerobically or otherwise, is a good thing, but each type of exercise serves a specific purpose. In the cases above, what was missing was lean muscle tissue. Nearly every female I have consulted responds to my advice to train with weights by saying: "I don't want to bulk up and look like a man." What a grave general misconception that is!

The absence of lean muscle tissue is the presence of fat and flab. Doing only cardio, walking, etc. will basically turn you into a smaller and still flabby (if not even flabbier) version of yourself. On the other hand, adding a few lb. of lean muscle tissue will in fact tighten the body. By doing only excessive amounts of aerobic exercise (treadmills, etc.) you may, in fact, cannibalize the very muscle tissue that you desperately need, which would be completely counter-productive to you reaching your goals.

"I CAN DO IT ALL MYSELF"

Most people think that by joining a gym and being shown the exercise machines, they will have all they need to hit the mark and get the body they so desperately want. This is, of course, utter nonsense. By way of analogy, let's assume I want to build a house. You (being a contractor or construction guru), plop me in the middle of all the equipment needed to build a house. Even if you were to show me what each piece of equipment is for, am I seriously going to be able to build a house? Not likely! It is a lot more specific and involved than that, isn't it? I would have to go to trade school or hire a teacher. Even after doing so, some form of apprenticeship would need to take place. Why on earth do people understand this when it comes to building a house, but not when it comes to building a body, which is immeasurably more complex and full of variables? They might search the Internet seeking the "magic-bullet" answer. Do I search the Internet on how to build a house? What do I get? Articles, pictures? Are you kidding me? Is that enough to get it done? Highly unlikely!

Back to "Martha." She decided to hire a trainer, one of my top coaches and she began to exercise properly. She came into the gym faithfully and always greeted me with a smile and repeatedly thanked me. We were saving her life, without a doubt. She began to lose weight…2, 10, 15, 20 lb. and so on. She got so excited with her progress that she wanted to see results even faster. My trainer named "Guy" (with nearly 20 years training experience) cautioned her to keep going slow and steady, but she woud not hear of it. She pushed way too hard and it wreaked havoc on her joints and circulatory system. Combined with a poor diet (she was not following the advice of our nutritionist), she lost her menstrual cycle, following that she developed blood clots in her legs. I have not seen or heard from Martha in over four months. Last I heard, she had been hospitalized and for all I know she could be dead.

People do indeed perish for lack of knowledge.
That is an extreme case, but it is one worth talking about.

A balanced exercise program and diet with the help of professionals is the way to go if you have little or no exercise/nutrition experience.

"I WANT TO LOSE THIS."

In my consultations, the previous phrase is usually accompanied by a finger pointing to the mid-section or gut. "My problem is here" (finger points again), most people say. I ask them "what about the rest of you then?"

"No, I am fine everywhere else. It's just my stomach," is usually the default reply.

Okay, let me get this straight: if your body fat is at 40 percent, you have joint issues, you walk like you are sitting at a desk and you are probably pre-diabetic, is the rest of you really *fine*? Not by a long shot. Health and well-being do not equate to just being skinny. The truth is that most people make losing weight their goal without giving even a second thought to being overall healthy and well. Is every skinny person you know in perfect health? No way. In fact, they may be in worse shape internally than someone who needs to lose 50 lb.!

Another analogy begs to be raised here. Let's say your house is sinking into its foundation, right into the ground, at its very core. Is repairing the windows going to fix that problem? Or is it just going to make it *look* a little better, prettier even? Likewise, the foundation of your body must be strong or you may wind up imploding, even if you *are* skinny.

The only way to reach your goals and maintain them long-term is to employ components of proper cardiovascular activity (consider what length, intensity, and heart rate) and weight training (doesn't have to be heavy) that is constantly progressive, along with a sensible eating plan. There you go. Save yourself some money, I just gave you the answer to the whole darn thing! Is it easy? No, it's not. It is no easier than building a house from scratch if you have never even held a hammer. You can, however, *learn* how to do both!

IT'S NOT ABOUT HOW SMART YOU ARE

I must confess to some degree of frustration here, please indulge me gentle reader.

Someone walks into my office and needs to lose 50 lb. Their posture looks like a bent wire coat hanger, they smoke a pack of cigarettes a day, and they have a knee problem. Then they tell me that they just want me to show them how to use the exercise machines. Am I on Candid Camera? This is a joke, right? You are talking about rewiring and recomposing the most complex organism on earth: a human body! We think nothing of spending thousands (rightfully so) on qualified contractors to fix our homes, or hundreds to have someone qualified to fix our cars. However, when it comes to fixing our bodies, "it's okay, I am going to do it myself." Am I the only one to whom that makes no sense, whatsoever?

You plan to undo ten years or more of physical abuse all by yourself since, after all, you *did* used to play football in college 20 years ago? NEWS FLASH! You may think you can still do that, but your body has kept on aging and it's going to get ugly if you go try out for an NFL team now, isn't it!

Nearly all my consultations included people who had no idea how to lose fat correctly and permanently. Over 85 percent of them had been on some sort of diet and I will say this here as well, not a single *one* managed to keep the fat off. It always came back. Why? It was done incorrectly, that's why. It was a desperate attempt to reverse years of bad habits and fix it all in a month by way of some pill, injection, or rabbit food diet. Is that reality? To some, it unfortunately is. It's all they know and all it equates to is a lack of knowledge.

Hold right there for a minute please. I always say this to my clients: "anything I say to you today is not because I think you are stupid, it is because I think you simply don't know how to go about this correctly. This is not a lack of *intelligence*, it is a lack of *knowledge*. There is a huge difference between the two."

The good book had it right: people perish for lack of knowledge. Oh boy, no kidding!

If I get in a race car at 200 mph and kill myself in the process, what exactly killed me, being stupid? No! Not knowing *how* to drive a car at that speed killed me; my lack of *knowledge* killed me.

It is no different in successful fat loss. Knowledge and application is all that is required. Having that knowledge along with the execution and implementation of that knowledge will yield results. Lawyers are brilliant. Are they all skinny and fit? Of course not! If it was all about brains, then some of us would be okay, but that isn't the case at all.

Get the proper information. Yes, *pay* someone the same way you would a contractor, plumber, or mechanic. How much does it cost? Each gym is different, but where I worked out of, we were able to get people help for much less than they expected to pay. Was it all the help they needed? In some cases, yes, and in others no. It is, however, better to get at least *some* information, than none at all.

I like to read about a great many things. A few years back, I had convinced myself that I could build a log home. What's the big deal, right? A few logs, nails, and a good whack of land is all that was needed. I even had friends in the construction industry who would rent me a backhoe. I read *dozens* of books and scoured the Internet on the matter. Guess what? I still live in a condo, but I still want that log home some day! Imagine if I had sat down and talked to just *one* person who had actually *done it* and built a log home. I would get more from that individual in a few minutes than I could ever get by reading reams of pages. Why? Well, he has actually *done it*! Likewise, if I want to learn to pilot an aircraft and I interview people who have read books about flying and I talk to one person who has actually flown for even 60 seconds, guess what? I am going to get more information from the person who has actually flown an aircraft before and has practical experience.

What's my point here? There is no shortage of information available online and in books, but is all of it viable? No, of course not.

You could argue here, "well I am reading *your* book, right, Marco?" Yes, you are! (Thank you for that, by the way.) The difference here is that you are dealing with material from someone who has actually done what you are looking to do, successfully. *Any* restrictive diet, *any* trainer can get you to lose 30 lb., in a month, but it will *never* last, period!

This is about lifestyle and consistency. Duct tape to fix a leaking roof will only act as a temporary Band-Aid type of cure, a short-term remedy. It will not fix the problem permanently. Likewise, a temporary restriction of your caloric intake through some type of "fad" low-cal diet will not fix things permanently. In fact, when you come off of that low calorie, no carb diet, what do you think will happen to you? Well, I can answer that from my experience as a trainer and consultant—you will gain it all back with interest!

Some of the people I trained came to me after having taken B5 and B12 vitamin injections with the intention of slowing the body's capability to process carbohydrates. However, in doing so they also drastically restricted their carbohydrate intake. They all lost a large amount of weight (muscle, fat, and water) and some of them also lost their hair, muscle tissue, and a lot of money as well! If you want to be lean and healthy for life, the only plan that will work is one that involves lifestyle.

PROGRESS IS A STEP BY STEP PROCESS

Boxing great Evander Holyfield routinely intimidated his opponents. He continued to do so well after most experts in the boxing world considered him to be "too old to fight and contend." Stand on the business end of one of his punches and you will get an idea, a very *painful* idea, of how wrong they were. Did Evander wake up one morning and just walk into a boxing ring as a great fighter? Obviously not. He had a lifetime of practice and a lifestyle that saw him take great strides to reach the pinnacle of success. This is the same case with NBA great Michael Jordan, tennis legend Bjorn Borg, or any other individual of prominence in any field. From Donald Trump to Reggie Jackson, the great race car driver Ayrton Senna to virtuoso character actor, Gary Oldman, each of these greats worked consistently to hone their skills. None of these people just "showed up" and had it happen for them, it took consistency and lifestyle.

The same things need to happen in order for successful fat loss to take place and then remain permanent. It is all about lifestyle. There are no quick changes that will last a lifetime.

Move!

Some people sit in their cars and actually (on occasion) turn their attention to driving. Some are busy (and I have actually seen this) yakking on cell phones, while they are shoving something down their throats, while the CD player is blasting, the personal DVD player is playing, and they are screaming at their kids. All of which is accomplished while travelling at speeds of over 100 km/hour. Speaking of which: Good Lord, I hope you are not reading this while you are supposed to be driving! (Get the audio book instead. It will be available soon!)

Some people have been at work all day sitting at a desk.

After they get home, they *sit* down for dinner and then after that it's, "Well, I'm tired, I think I'll *sit* and relax for a bit."

We now live in a day and age where "walking" is considered exercise. Let me say that again. The whole notion of walking is no longer regarded as a primary means of getting from here to there—we have cars for that. Walking is now considered exercise! *Walking* is almost treated like "a great new idea" to lose weight!

Think about it; those of us who workout at a gym get into a car and *drive* to a gym so we can *walk* on a treadmill. We build expensive machines to walk and run on with the primary focus being to lose weight. I hear you out there, gentle reader. You might be saying, "this guy is nuts, I can't *walk* everywhere!" Since I frequently travel on business by car and airplane, it is safe to say "you are preaching to the choir." I am not saying it is possible to walk *everywhere*, but I am asking if you walk *at all*.

THE "GYM" ALL AROUND YOU

Where are you as you read this at this very moment? On a subway, bus, plane, or perhaps seated comfortably in an easy chair? Do something for me, please? Stand up if you are sitting or sit down if you are standing. Congratulations! You have just performed an exercise whose movement worked over 300 different muscles. It's called a squat. Cool, huh? Go ahead, do it again, I dare you. What's that, you feel "silly" you say? How silly will you feel when a few years from now you might be walking around in pain (if at all) thanks to atrophy (stiff muscles) because you didn't take the time to simply move now? Okay, that is a bit extreme, but we are dealing with an extremely important issue, my friends.

Now, I am not going to turn this into an in-depth exercise book; there are reams of books already available on that subject. There are, however, some basic principles we need to grasp about exercise in order to get us started on the right foot. (One moment please, while I get a coffee. Yes, I still drink coffee!)

Okay, I am back. Thank you for waiting.

SOME BASICS

In lifting weights, the fastest way possible to trigger fat loss through exercise is by working the biggest muscle groups we have, namely the legs and back. These two muscle groups account for as much as 80% of your total body mass. I want to pause here for a moment to say that I believe from experience that an exercise program that includes all

muscle groups is necessary to achieve both optimal fitness and symmetry. We don't want to walk around with legs like watermelons and arms looking like spaghetti. (By the way, I also eat spaghetti! It's a carb. I know! I am Italian!)

Having said that, the main focus of this book is to equip you with the basics of fat loss and a healthy lifestyle. There is an abundance of exercise books you can buy to learn about bodybuilding and different workout programs. But for now, back to "Exercise 101," if you will.

SHOP BY PHONE FITNESS

Let me dispel a myth that has been made famous by selling expensive machines to people late at night as they sit and chow down on junk-food. Yes, you know what I'm talking about...I am talking about the dreaded "infomercial." The staging of this work of fiction requires more suspension of disbelief than a sci-fi movie. Here we see a group of muscle bound guys with "washboard" abs that you could grind the gunk off your dirty socks on (gross) or use to crack walnuts. By the way, they are all "movie star" good looking with perfect hair. Hey wait! They are starting to look a lot like those people from the beer and junk-food commercials we talked about... maybe it's the *same* people? Ridiculous.

"ABS"-OLUTELY NOT

Then we have the Barbie types on these infomercials. Again now, let me pause to make a point...I admire these people. They are in the shape they are because they take care of themselves, exercise, and eat right, nothing negative at all for me to say here. What is, however, completely absurd is the idea that "now you too can look like this" by simply buying this "ab thing" or "thigh thing" and using it for just 15 minutes a day! Check with any legitimate health professional or trainer you can pull out of the phone book. If they are honest and knowledgeable, they will tell you that it is next to basically *impossible* to lose even an ounce of fat by working your abs and doing sit-ups.

Earlier, I spoke about targeting the biggest muscle groups on your body to speed fat loss...abs are some of the smallest. To give you an idea of size, we are talking roughly the same size as strips of bacon here. To activate a muscle and generate enough heat for these "strips" to actually burn off significant fat is genetically impossible. Don't believe me? Go ahead then, take the next year and do an hour of ab crunches (modified sit-us) per day and see what happens...you will be right where you started as far as fat in your mid-section is concerned. You might actually get your ab muscles to stick out and make you look even heavier or herniated!

On a personal note, I remember walking into a gym when I weighed well over 300 lb. and sporting size 54 pants. Let me tell you *exactly* what went through my head as I passed by the ultra-fit people around me. "Right, I am gonna lie down like a beached whale, my gut flopping from side to side and do ab crunches." Tell ya what, when I *did* find the energy to actually drop to the ground, the next things on my mind were: How am I going to not have my shirt pull up and expose my gut to the masses as I (ahem) "crunch"? Followed by, how in blazes am I ever going to be able to get back up again? Which logically led to, I am starving, what's for lunch?

There *are* significant benefits to working out your abs and they *absolutely should* be worked on, but the right way and for the right reasons. Working out your abs will strengthen your "core," these are the muscles located in the middle (or at the "core") of your body (both back and front) and that is a good thing. You can perhaps make your abs more defined in the long run, but you will only be able to do it if you get rid of the fat that is in front, between, and possibly behind them.

CROSS TRAINING

In order to effectively burn fat and keep your body progressing, I suggest you look into cross-training or interval training. There is a bevy of books available on the subject.

In short, you will be targeting a lot of different muscle groups at once (these are called "compound exercises"). These exercises hit as many muscles as possible at once and will help you achieve the most effective results. This type of training keeps your heart rate elevated, while working with weights. It really is one of the best ways to burn fat.

Stay away from tangents. By this, I mean the new "Abs this," or "Abs that," contraption. Be realistic! Remember, if you have 35 inch legs, that ab device will do you no good. Strike at the heart of matters and blast the entire body!

Ignorance is potentially fatal. Even if it's not fatal it will surely cost us in some way. We need to educate ourselves and become knowledgeable on matters such as food and weight loss for ourselves. We cannot blindly believe what some major diet and fitness food manufacturers, natural herbal remedy, supplement groups, exercise machine manufacturers, and weight loss corporations are telling us. We need to get the goods on our own. Remember, they are in this as corporations trying to make money. There is nothing wrong with making money, but ignorance and indifference should not be what lines their pockets.

It is indeed *caveat emptor*—buyer beware.

Starving to be Fat

One of the things that I could not understand when I was at my heaviest weight was that I was hardly eating and yet I was still huge. I wondered how it was possible to skip breakfast (I never was a "breakfast" person), maybe have lunch, and then just eat around dinner and yet still be fat. It served as an interesting premise as I set out to research various caloric restriction diets when I finally decided that I was going to try to lose my blubber.

"I barely eat, yet I am fat and I keep *gaining* weight!"

Well, I figured at that point that there would be no point in going on a super low calorie diet, since in essence and without trying I was already kind of on one. Barely eating meant gaining weight, how could this be possible? I decided then that there had to be another way or at least an explanation. After exhaustive reading and self-education, I developed an analogy that might help us understand this better.

STORED ENERGY

Let's assume for a moment that someone commits a crime (shame on them) and they are in jail in some far off country. In the morning, the guard comes by with a small amount of food and the prisoner eats it. Hours pass and there is no more food to be found. So the prisoner begins to think, "hey, are they ever going to feed me again today? I am starving here!" (You see? Crime does not pay!)

Well, though the person is in jail, they still do have a brain to reason with. The next day, the same thing happens. A little bit of food in the morning, but this time the prisoner stops to think: "I remember what happened yesterday; no food came for hours and I nearly starved! Today I am going to save some of this food and store it, so as not to run out of energy later."

So our inmate digs a secret little hole in his cell and he begins storing food. Storing, because he is afraid he will run out of food or energy later.

NEWSFLASH! That is exactly how your body works!

Okay reader, here is your get-out-of-jail-free card, back to reality now.

The excess fat you are carrying can also be called "stored energy." What you are carrying is energy that is not being used and that results in fat. Why is that energy still there, even though you are not eating all that much? Simply put, you are "starving to be fat." You have told your body by way of your lifestyle that your current weight and body fat percentage are normal for you as well as "healthy." You defined this by skipping meals and restricting calories. How? (Good question!) When you set out to lose that fat (stored energy), your body views it as a threat to your well-being. In essence, you are asking your body to lose that excess energy and your body is coming back at you saying "I refuse." The body continues, "I refuse to give up this stored energy because you are not giving me enough energy in the first place. Why on earth would I let go of what you have on you if I feel you are not giving me enough to begin with? No way, buddy, I am going to make sure I store every little bit I get, 'cus I need it!"

Make sense? Let's go a little further with this example. Since your lifestyle has defined that your current weight and body fat percentage are "normal" for you, it will view any attempt you make to lose that stored energy as a threat. It will erect a wall of protection called "body fat" and will do all it can to "save" you. It is designed to do so and it is just doing its job. Did a lightbulb just go on in your mind?

I was starving and I yet was huge because I was forcing my body to store energy due to the lack of energy coming in. WOW!

Back to jail for a second. (Relax a Navy SEAL team will be here to get you out of there in a minute.)

If our prisoner were to be incarcerated in a more "civilized" jail, (now there's an oxymoronic term if I have ever heard one) and he knew that there was food coming in at regular intervals, there would be no reason for him to store that food (energy) in the first place and save it for later. He'd just eat it, since he knew there would be a consistent supply of it.

(Okay, hear the choppers? The SEAL team has arrived and rescued you. Ah, freedom!)

Your body would behave exactly the same way. It would recognize that there would be more energy coming in throughout the course of the day and therefore it would not feel the need to stow any extra energy other than what it needs to function.

You have given your body a schedule and, as a result, it is expecting either to starve or to not starve.

Feed it!

MEAL FREQUENCY

I ate my way to fat loss by furnishing my body with five to six smaller meals and snacks throughout the day. It has no choice but to let go of any energy and not store it, simply because I have taught it that I will not starve it. As a result, my body "likes" me and will gladly release any excess energy since it does not feel the need to hold onto anything more than it needs. When I pair that approach with exercise, any unnecessarily large amount of stored energy has no chance; it *has* to go so my body can relax, it knows it will be fed.

"What? He eats six times a day?"

Relax! I am not gorging on junk food and buckets of fried chicken here! I eat wholesome and real foods. Veggies, poultry, the right fats and carbs. (Since I did not set out to write a specific diet book, please go out and buy *The Abs Diet* by the editor of *Men's Health* Magazine. It has a great primer course on healthy foods and meal frequency. Why reinvent the wheel? These guys nailed it!)

By *not* eating enough, your body will do all it can to cling to everything you put in your mouth and store it, because it fears you will never give it enough energy to survive. It thinks you are in some far off jail or marooned on a deserted island, neither of which have a food supply readily available.

You can give your body a good schedule or a bad one. Either way you choose to go, it will react and adapt to what you have taught it are normal conditions.

How many calories do you need? I have no idea and any diet that says it does know (without first having sat down and analyzed how your particular body makes use of its calories), should be treated as suspect!

Susan, the Last Thing I Ever Expected.

In 2006 when I attended a course to certify as a Personal Trainer Specialist I met a lady who caught the attention of the entire room. At first, it was because she arrived late and disrupted the class, but later on she commanded attention for other reasons.

Susan epitomized "fitness." She was 38-years-old and had the appearance of someone ten years her junior, and she still does. At her suggestion, an email list was circulated among all of the students so we could write each other and compare notes prior to taking the exam. Susan and I wound up writing each other and decided to get together to help each other study, well actually...more like CRAM!

At the time, Susan was married and our brief friendship was fuelled strictly by the need to study and pass the exam! She assumed I was intelligent and I also assumed that she was intelligent and must have know all there was to know about fitness. I thought she would be a great choice to help me pass the exam. I guess we were both at least partially right, as we did wind up passing.

On the first evening we got together, we cracked open the textbooks and settled into the business at hand. She had heard brief highlights about my weight loss, as I had shared them with the class, and asked me to further expand on my journey that evening, which I did.

Now remember, way back in this book I had mentioned the "memory" of fat? Even though I had lost the extra pounds successfully, that I still at times "felt" fat, the term for which is "dysmorphia." By the time Susan and I met, I was no longer married and had been separated for years. But I noticed something interesting. Eventhough Susan had what a lot of people would call "a perfect physique," she had personal challenges that had nothing to do with anything of a physical nature. You can read more about Susan in her contributing chapter "Poise and Power: My Personal Chapter on Fitness."

"What? You mean gorgeous people with incredible physiques have other issues just like I do? Man, I would give anything to have abs like that!"

Or would you? Few know what it takes and for those who do know, few are willing to pay the price. Excellence does not happen overnight. Ask Michael Jordan, who couldn't sink a basket if his life depended on it when he first started, if it came easily to him.

People made assumptions about me when I was fat and they made assumptions about Susan, who was a National Fitness title holder. Ironic, to say the least. Her vulnerability inspired me and made me think anything was possible, as I listened to her speak of some of her challenges.

I do remember thinking that if I ever ran into someone this fit, pretty and also single, that there would be no way they would ever be interested in me. Again, the memory of fat was taking its toll on me, even then, years after regaining control of my life.

In any event, after Susan and I passed the exam, we fell out of touch for some time. I moved on with my life and she moved ahead with hers, we occasionally wrote each other to touch base, but that was it.

Well, that was it until Susan had felt the need to make changes in her life and separated from her husband. After a while, and completely unexpectedly, we got back in touch and had dinner. I was happy that I was going to see my friend again, but I was so nervous! Even Susan doesn't know to this day the amount of gut sucking I did in front of the mirror, hours before we met. It wasn't because I had feelings for her, or that I considered our dinner a "date"; it was because I went through that ritual any time I had to get dressed to go out. Yup, all this even after having lost well over 100 lb. and by most people's accounts, looking decent. We caught up and reminisced about the silly exam pressures, etc. For some time after that, we exchanged emails and began calling each other more frequently and a deeper friendship was formed.

After some time, Susan confessed to having feelings for me. A total dream for a former fat guy, right? Think about it: former fat guy lands fitness babe! It's the stuff of movies! Well, it wasn't a dream at all, in fact it was terrifying for me.

The very instant she first told me that she loved me, I felt as if the 140 lb. I had lost somehow came back and attached itself to my body.

Of course I was elated, as well as terrified! I was also in the midst of some other personal plans that made the timing seem not quite right, but I also had a whack of excuses (about 140 lb. of them) as to why she and I would never be anything other than friends.

Susan persisted. She continued to tell me she loved me, even when I could not say I felt the same way for her. She had incredible courage and purity of heart. There is no way she could understand the battle I was waging with fat, even years after I had been victorious.

The thoughts ran something like; "There is no way that a woman who looks like this could ever be interested in you long-term. People like you don't get the gorgeous girls, people like you get the ones looking for comfort, or for a shoulder to cry on. Are you nuts, man? This woman could get anyone she wants! It must be a rebound on her part, yeah, that's what this must be. Give it some time and it will pass!"

It never *did* pass! She kept coming on like a freight train! Finally, long after my feelings towards her had changed, I gave into this beautiful woman. I took a chance. We both did.

Nearly three years later, we are happier than we ever dreamed we could be.

I wish I could say that all my mental "weight" issues have been resolved, but that would be a lie. Susan has been magnificent in building my confidence and has even let me train her at the gym. What an incredible experience!

I remember the day that she won her second FAME National Championship, we walked around the venue checking out sponsors, etc. Susan put on a sweater and I said "honey, you worked hard, lose the sweater, and show off your incredible physique, you deserve it!" I am so glad I did that, but let me tell you, as we walked around that place with all eyes (rightfully) on her, I tried hard to not think that they were then looking at me and saying: "Wow, what's a babe like that doing with a guy like him?"

"MEMORY OF FAT" REFUSED TO DEVELOP AMNESIA.

As recently as a few weeks ago she said, "Honey, you need to stop wearing your fat clothes. They no longer fit and you are no longer that man." Once again, I resisted. I clung to clothes that were comfortable and baggy. I didn't realize how much heavier they made me look!

About one month ago we were out shopping and I spotted a really nice pair of jeans, but they were a size 36. I hadn't been a 36 in over 20 years!

Susan: "Try these on, hon."

Marco (sarcastically): "Yeah, right!"

Susan (to the sales person): "Excuse me, Miss. What size pants do you think would fit this man?"

"About a 36," she offers.

Susan gives me the quintessential "told ya so" kind of look. She stands all of 5 ft. 1 and change, but inside she is 9 feet tall.

So I yielded and, yup, they fit!

I walked out of the change room wearing the pants. Susan gave me a high five and said "Congratulations, baby! I am so proud of you. What an achievement!"

I still have the size tag from the pants!

Think I have bought a new wardrobe yet?

Think Susan has stopped bugging me to go out and buy new clothes, that are not "fat guy" clothes?

The answer is yes to the former, and no to the latter! But I resisted buying new clothes for years!

Think I have bent over to tie my running shoes much in the last few years? Nope. I only do it if the laces come undone. Am I able to bend over and do so? Of course, but for years I could not and that memory, that natural reflex, is still there.

THERE ARE STILL SOME INSECURITIES

"Fat guy fears" are still there. The amount of attention Susan (deservedly) gets, when she is training, as a result of her modelling, or just standing there looking gorgeous, can test the resolve and security of most any man. I confess, I fight it still, but she does all she can to make me feel as safe and secure as possible. The rest is up to me! If you love and believe in someone and you want to help them advance in life, you must put them in front of your own needs, and not put your fears ahead of them.

I have accompanied Susan to and directed all of her modelling photo shoots. I see her under lights and in print and think to myself "you have *got* to be *kidding* me! What are you doing with a guy like me?"

Then there is the equalizer. With all of the accolades she has rightfully received as an elite fitness persona, she reminds me of her own struggles... and asks me the same question.

For more information and images of both Susan and I, please visit her website; www.seriouscurvestraining.com

"Poise and Power"
A Personal View on Fitness
by Susan Braumberger-Arruda (3 Time Figure Champion)

With over 25 years of training and with numerous fitness titles, I'm privileged and thankful to be able to contribute some of my own thoughts and personal experiences and to offer a different perspective on food, exercise, and a healthy lifestyle. I felt excited, as well as intimidated and slightly overwhelmed to write a chapter based on my own personal experiences and thoughts on such matters. To encapsulate a lifetime of experience and knowledge effectively and concisely into a chapter is quite a task, especially when the man I'm with possesses the gift of eloquent expression.

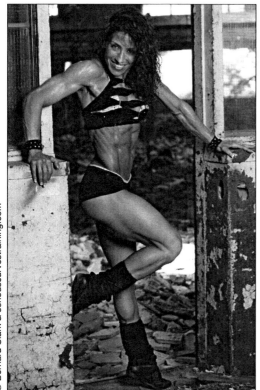

BODY IMAGE

To begin, I will address body image. The most common misconception and assumption people make about me upon first glance is that I'm a confident woman who has it all together. Until about 2007 nothing could have been further from the truth. The personal challenges I faced were massive and very real and resulted in me having an extremely low self-esteem, despite the image of fitness that was clearly portrayed when people looked at me. (We all have our areas of struggle.) When a person looks good on the exterior, the default assumption is that the person is happy and "has it all." This is obviously not the case. Without even having to name names, I'm sure that certain celebrities and famous pop stars will instantly come to mind to validate my point. The fact of the matter is that often those who look so together on the outside may indeed have enormous insecurities, issues, and distorted body images that do not match what is noticeable at first glance. No doubt about it, I am thankful that I turned to fitness training and exercise as a positive outlet, but I also found out over time and over the course of my life that physical fitness alone, certainly isn't the complete answer to being happy.

THE BALANCING ACT

We must continually strive for a balance in all areas of our lives. Everyone's life should encompass the power of positive thinking, spirituality (my own relationship with God has been instrumental in my recent life altering changes; it only took me 20 plus years, better late than never!) healthy balanced eating, adequate rest, and exercise. As a mother of two teens, I fully understand how difficult keeping it all in balance really is. At times, maintaining a balance may not be possible due to circumstances in life, but overall, that is what we must continually strive to achieve, nonetheless.

A healthy body image certainly begins in the mind. Thinking that you will be happy upon reaching an ideal weight or look is inaccurate. In having a perfectionist attitude, I constantly strived for more and better, but it never proved to be enough. I had to finally make peace with that fact and change my outlook and ideals. Placing unrealistic and overwhelming expectations on ourselves can be disastrous, disappointing, and can even result in severe depression. More does not always equate to better or happier. I immersed myself in training as an outlet for escape and as a coping mechanism. In the midst of that, I also battled with keeping food consumption at bay and my weight in balance (although again, to look at me, no one would have ever guessed).

One of my saving graces became weight training as it served to shift my focus from the scale to the mirror. I realized that body composition (total fat vs. total lean muscle) was a more accurate measurement of health and leanness. We can become so preoccupied with the numbers that appear on the scale that it can wreck our mindset, mood, and attitude. The degree of error in an every day scale measurement is substantial. It does not factor good lean muscle weight vs. fat, hydration levels, or the effects of the monthly female cycle as it pertains to water retention, etc. If you're a slave to the scale, throw it out and develop a healthier method of staying on target; take measurements on a monthly basis and use your mirror as your guide on a daily basis.

BALANCING FOOD CHOICES

Eating healthy, making good food choices, and keeping food intake in balance is one of life's greatest ongoing challenges. What is that balance? Well, it is different for everybody. Is one tool right for every job? Of course not! You cannot approach weight loss by making temporary changes for a limited time and expect anything to stick. Logically, this cannot work. Portion control becomes a major issue when we consider stress eating, so keeping a healthy perspective on eating is critical for success. I've gone through bouts of compulsive overeating and that "throwing in the towel" defeatist attitude which is most destructive to finding a balance and will only cause further negativity towards ourselves. Never give up when this happens, for we all stumble and fall. Be forgiving with yourself and stay stubbornly determined.

You must consider eating with a common sense approach that is most realistic to your life. If you absolutely love chocolate and know it is your downfall, to try to completely restrict it forever is ludicrous and unrealistic. Sure you're going to have days when you overeat and indulge more than you should with certain foods, but allow yourself some flexibility and engage in positive self-talk. If you tell yourself this is the very last time you will allow yourself to eat a certain food, then of course you'll want to eat more than you normally would and you will most certainly end up overindulging. Instead, tell yourself, "Yeah, I know I've messed up. I'll allow myself to eat some and know that I can have it again in the near future." If you don't gorge, you're less likely to give up entirely. Make adjustments accordingly. Balance such temporary setbacks by doing a little more training the very next day in combination with getting back to healthy eating. Don't just give up and sabotage all your efforts because you caved or "fell off the wagon." Don't get *on* a wagon, just get back to balanced eating, asap! *Be forgiving as well as disciplined with yourself.*

The plus side of setbacks is that in changing things up, both in the way you eat and train, keeps your body guessing. Your body is forced to make thermal adjustments to account for the unexpected changes and on a positive note, doesn't develop a rigid "set point." I have put this into practice more times than I can dare to count. Be forgiving with yourself, yet remain persistent. The overindulgence does not come without a price to pay. Simply pay it and move on.

CONSTANT PROGRESS

In order for training to be progressive, it should always change to yield results. After several weeks of doing the same exercises or following the same scheduled program, the body brilliantly adapts to what we're doing. This is often referred to as a plateau. We have to outsmart it to prompt and elicit further changes. When you experience that stubborn dilemma where your body's progress seems to come to a grinding halt, you need to respond by changing things up in some way. Variety is truly the spice of life and is a required and vital component for consistent progress. Upon starting any active program, progress is noticeable and can occur quickly and steadily (although it never seems quick enough). Changes are more rapid in the beginning and, over time, they gradually taper off and may cease. This is a temporary predicament which requires change and creativity. Make changes and adjustments to either your exercise program, your diet, or ideally, both. Outsmart and be more stubborn than your fat. Conviction and persistence pay off big time in this area and you must have resolve to see results. When you reach one of these plateaus you should probably consider a consultation with a pro, if you haven't already.

Train regularly and incorporate many varying elements of fitness training into your workouts. Training seriously for 30-60 minutes is far better than spending two and a half hours at the gym. Socializing and training do not go together. Time is of the essence and there never seems to be enough of it, so make the absolute most of it. Shorter sessions can also be viewed with less dread. Train seriously, stay focused throughout your workout to get your heart rate up and keep it elevated.

FLEX APPEAL

One of the most common questions people ask me about training revolves around flexibility. "How did you get so flexible?" they will often ask. I worked extremely hard to gain flexibility and even harder to keep it. You can't let up and neglect it or you'll lose it. This component of fitness is the absolute hardest to get back, especially as you age! I didn't have the advantage of any type of formal training (like gymnastics, which people often assume). I've met many who did have the privilege of training and have lost their gains. The sad fact is if you don't use it, you lose it and if you've got it, you must consistently work hard to maintain it! It all goes in a heartbeat; there's no justice here, folks. I stretch religiously and incorporate it throughout all my workouts. If you've just worked a muscle in a set and it's tight, then you should stretch it. It's a simple common sense approach. This also helps to minimize and prevent injuries, as well as muscular imbalances. We all need a minimum level of flexibility to be able to perform functions of daily living. I work as an aquatics instructor and educator in a Toronto middle school. It's alarming when I come across students of 11 to 14 years of age who don't have basic flexibility. Flexibility is a component and requirement for healthy bodies with a normal range of motion. When I was their age, I recall watching T.V. positioned in the side splits; a little extreme, perhaps, but doable, nonetheless.

STANDING TALL

Implement simple training techniques into your everyday life. Besides walking more and taking the stairs, take heed of your posture and sit upright. This is another basic area that is shocking and not up to par in young students, as well as adults. This is especially visible when watching students sitting on the ground with no back support to rely on. Using your muscles to sit upright requires conscious muscular effort and control.

How you carry yourself makes a non-verbal statement, not only about your level of physical fitness, but your confidence level as well. In teaching the importance and validity of this point, I present the scenario of two students or individuals who have applied for a position and attend the same interview. Let's say that all things factor evenly and it's pretty close—an even race. However, one individual has rounded stooped shoulders and a slouched postural position in the interview while the other individual has perfect, upright posture, while either seated or standing. Who do you think would get the job? Well, it would more than likely be the indiviual with the edge; the person with the better posture.

THE FORMULA FOR GOOD POSTURE

With that being said, let's address the recipe for better posture:
Push your shoulders down and back (depress and retract), align your shoulders over your hips and slightly tilt your hips forward and engage your abdominals by contracting and tightening your muscles by con-

sciously pulling your stomach in tight. Aim to line up your shoulders over your hips. Visualize being able to keep an invisible cup of water positioned on top of your head. (you may actually want to try that as a little test). At first it may feel completely unnatural if you are not accustomed to that position or stance, but over time, and with regular consistent practice, it will begin to feel more natural and become second nature. Take small steps and start with personal awareness.

"I AM PREGNANT, SO I CAN'T TRAIN"

Training and pregnancy is a fitness combination that tends to raise automatic apprehension and confusion. Your doctor may not be very helpful here and, for liability reasons, may provide you with very little instruction and direction, as I learned firsthand. Assuming you are healthy and have no high risk pregnancy factors, you can and should continue to do what you were doing prior to getting pregnant, but while being very diligent about listening to your body. Acute, sharp pains of any kind always indicate that you should stop immediately (whether you are pregnant or not)! Make adjustments throughout your pregnancy; they're necessary and required. I don't recommend high impact sports, especially once you start to put on additional weight. If you're an avid runner, move the sport into the water. Attach yourself to a tether strap or take a specifically targeted aqua fitness class. The water is an incredibly safe and beneficial training environment, which is often misunderstood or overlooked. Make constant changes as required, but keep moving. I trained right until the day prior to delivery. After my first trimester, abdominal crunches no longer felt right, nor did decline bench work.

THE RELAXIN HORMONE

Nope. It's not the relaxing hormone, it's the relaxin hormone. Although, relaxation of certain joints has a lot to do with this unique hormone. The relaxin hormone is produced and secreted by the ovalries druing pregnanc, to assist in the birthing process. It does this by enabling additional expansion and flexbility of the cervical and pelvic muscles. However, this added elasticity and flexibility is not exclusive to those areas, but in fact all joints and ligaments. Though this is a wonderful added benefit, it does present some unique challenges, and perhaps even some unfavorable consequences for the elite athlete. In essence, there is no "off" switch. The usual range of motion can be easily overextended and injury can result.

Be in tune with your body, make adjustments and eliminate exercises that do not feel quite right. In the last trimester be cautious of the relaxin hormone and hold back with respect to flexibility and ballistic movements of any kind. The hormone is not specific to the area for which it is targeted and hits all the joints and can consequently, produce some joint instability.

"I'M EATING FOR TWO"

No actually, you're not.

Do not use pregnancy as an excuse not to train and to eat for two. Eating for two is just an excuse to overeat. If you think that way, you will be doomed! Don't deprive yourself either; just eat healthy and keep portion sizes under control. Otherwise, you will gain more weight than you should or than you need to and consequently, will develop stretch marks and not feel good about yourself as a result of the excess weight gain. Think about this rationally: Your baby will not (in most cases) weigh more than 10 1b. Factor in the placenta at 4-6 lb. and perhaps 5 lb. of water weight and you're at 20 lb. I gained 18–20 lb. for both my pregnancies and gave natural childbirth to two healthy babies. I'm not a doctor nor am I attempting to dispense medical advice. This is just my personal training philosophy with respect to my own real life experiences in pregnancy and it worked for me.

WOMEN, WEIGHTS AND "BULKING UP"

Women often have a misconception about training with weights. "I don't want to bulk up or put on big muscles." Well, very few women desire that look, nor is it possible for many females to achieve it. Your body type comes into consideration here. Upon first glance, people assume I lift and train with heavy weights, but I do not. However, I did spend quite a few of my earlier years lifting to acquire mass. In later years I worked to sculpt and fine tune my muscles and my overall physique in order to create symmetry. I currently train with light weights and higher repetitions (10–20 or more reps depending on the muscle being worked) and I often work with no loads at all, just my body weight. (Again folks, keep in mind that I've been training a lifetime and if you are beginning a fitness program with the goal of ultimately losing 50 lb. or more, the focus must be different in order to yield results and stay injury free.)

Women do not pack on muscle easily unless they partake in steroid use—this is a fact. They simply do not have the testosterone that is required to naturally do so. Put your minds at ease and realize that it just will not happen! I worked incredibly hard for the shape and muscles I have developed and it's all completely natural. I have never, ever compromised or felt tempted to do so. Steroids have never been an option for me. Remember, I've been training for a very long time, so I have achieved muscle density along with muscle memory and I've always been committed to being physically active and fit. Your personal trainer should help you devise the right training program to achieve the results and goals you desire. Natural muscle equates to a toned and sexy physique that enables your body to not only look better, but allows your body to function more efficiently and burn more calories at rest.

As I have already mentioned, for the most part I train with light weights and strict form. Yes, there are many, many training principles and techniques, but too many people exercise with improper form and weights that are far heavier than they can properly lift. This can certainly lead to injuries. This practice also does not allow you to target the intended muscle for the specific exercise, which means you're wasting your time doing it incorrectly. That's a lot of energy and hard work dispensed for no good reason and no positive outcome!

Start with developing fundamentals (using your own body weight) and work from there. Knowledge and proper instruction are vital components for success and continued progress. I train to look and feel good all the time, not just for a competition. I only began to hit the stage three years ago. Competition has never been my main focus for training hard, so I manage to look pretty consistent year round. Training is a lifestyle for me and I strive to achieve my personal best on a consistent and regular basis. Sure, I'll make changes to my eating a month prior to a show, but I don't go through radical changes because that's not what it's all about for me. Competing serves to inspire me and enables me to set goals. Competition keeps me striving to further improve on my personal best. Make training and exercise realistic for your lifestyle. Radical changes are not natural, nor healthy for your body.

REASONS WHY WE TRAIN

Too many people cannot pull or push up their own body weight which is something I consider to be a bare essential safety skill requirement. A single pull up can have the ability to save your life in a life or death situation. I've encountered many students and individuals who cannot pull themselves back up into a canoe from within the water in ideal conditions (indoor, with no wind or rough water or terrain). This fact is alarming and a cause for concern. Great looking abs may look sexy, but they won't save you in a situation such as this one. However, training for strength will.

The bottom line is that we may all have different reasons for beginning an exercise program, but, generally, we all want to look, as well as feel good, and certainly not at the expense of our health. We need to have all these elements in balance. Tackle exercise and eating with a sane, life-long approach that is conducive to your lifestyle and make it doable and pleasant. I've gone through my share of highs and lows when it comes to exercise. There have been long periods I endured through where I dreaded training, but developed the mental tenacity to do it anyway. At times, I viewed it as a chore that just had to be done despite how I felt. It was not easy, that's for sure, but it was a definite requirement for my personal fitness success and my mental well-being. Try to incorporate activities you enjoy and change things up regularly to alleviate boredom and stagnation. Exercise and health are not a destination, but a journey with peaks and valleys. Remain open-minded, get in tune to your body, and stay positive. Always delight in the gift of movement.

Being happy certainly encompasses many things. I'm so grateful for having met Marco and finding true love. Following the principles of taking it slowly to ensure success (much like fitness), we first developed a friendship, followed by a deep, meaningful relationship in which we are both continuously growing and enjoying life to the fullest. I now also recognize that being with the right person can certainly help an individual achieve maximum potential and growth, personal confidence, and joy. I certainly wish everyone the courage required to take the first small steps in fitness to be followed by great successes in their personal growth and progress! Keep the faith and persevere in all challenging areas in life and make efforts to find joy in all that you do.

With poise and power,
Susan Braumberger-Arruda

You can visit Susan's website at: www.seriouscurvestraining.com

Small Changes, Big Results.

When I was in New York acting as music director for the musical, *The Count of Monte Cristo* I found myself in a city whose rush-hour traffic is as famous as its Broadway musicals. Actually, *every* hour of the day seemed like rush hour in New York. One of my favourite pastimes while I was there was to stand at the intersection nearest to our rental apartment and count. What was I counting? (I am glad you asked.) I was counting the number of actual "civilian owned" (anything that was not a cab, a limo, or a bus) vehicles on the busy stretch near Times Square. I was curious as to how many private cars I might see stopped at a red light at one time. The highest count I recorded was a grand total of seven "everyday" cars. Everything else was either checkered black or yellow, or had four more doors and was six feet longer than any normal car.

THE TORTOISE AND THE HARE

During my two months in "the Big Apple" there were several meetings with directors, agents, and actors etc. In order to get to those meetings, we would leave our apartment at West 51st and 7th and pile into one of those same checkered cabs I'd spent time counting. After two or three such trips, I noticed something; we'd be sitting in a cab and a pedestrian who might have been a few blocks back would pass us over and over again at nearly every intersection. I thought to myself, "what the heck am I doing? I am sitting here like a fat cat, spending untold amounts of money and that guy is getting there faster than I am, and free of charge!" In New York City, walking or riding a bicycle was faster than motorized transit, so I suggested that we consider walking on our next trip. From that point on we walked nearly every day to each of our meetings. This meant, thirst! I substituted my cola, alternating instead between water and orange juice. We might walk 20–30 minutes each day if not more and this went on for nearly two months. Before I knew it, the pants I had bought prior to making the trip to NYC no longer fit—they were looser. I thought this was incredible. What other changes had I made? Why was this happening? I still had not even *seen* a treadmill up close or picked up a dumbbell. I had not educated myself in any way about nutrition or weight loss...but I had lost weight and it was noticeable. I was becoming paranoid as to how I was going to keep this weight loss up once I got back to Toronto.

All told, after almost eight weeks I was in New York, I came back to Toronto a staggering 30 lb. lighter.

Now, a word of caution here. That is an extreme amount of weight to lose in such a short period of time. The reason this happened was that I had been completely inactive for years prior to my time in NYC and the majority of the weight that I lost was "water weight" (I didn't even know what that was back then). I can tell you now that "water weight" has to do with the amount of water our bodies store. For years, I had not been moving much at all and I was also dehydrated. You don't have to feel thirsty for your body to be in a dehydrated state. It all happens when we do not drink enough water (in particular) and our bodies hang on for dear life to the water that is already in our system just to survive. Since I began re-hydrating (by drinking on those long walks), this allowed my body to rid itself of moisture and water "trapped" in my body. Pick up a jug of water and you'll notice—it's heavy. Imagine that amount of weight being purged from your body and you'll begin to have a sense of the dramatic effect water weight loss will have on a body.

GET OFF THE COUCH

The main point I am making here is that we need to *move*. If you have been sedentary and have not performed any type of sustained movement such as walking, and you finally begin to move, your body will go into the best kind of "shock" possible and it will react. It will react positively and the benefits to your overall health will materialize almost instantly, whether you notice this happening or not.

My New York City experience had removed a large part of physical inactivity and dehydration from my life. These two had been replaced by walking (which I had no clue actually meant *exercise*) and water which re-hydrated my body without me even knowing it. Remember, I began drinking water on my walks in the city *not* because I was trying to lose weight, but just because I was thirsty.

As my return to Toronto approached, that paranoia I had mentioned earlier began to vanish. The simple truth was that I could take both of these "accidental" weight loss changes to my lifestyle and make them *deliberate* parts of my life in Toronto.

From that moment on, the weight I had begun to lose in NYC never came back. When I returned home friends and family were stunned by my appearance, I really liked that feeling. When someone is as overweight as I was, the first time you hear the words "hey, you lost weight," is similar to winning the lottery. The motivation you feel surges and you want to keep going. For me, it was the first time in my life that I dared to believe that I *could* lose all that fat and, hopefully, keep it off and so I determined I was going to do just that. Indeed, that weight has never come back, nor will it ever.

TO SUM IT ALL UP

I made small changes, resulting in big time fat loss, and I didn't even *know* that these changes would cause that loss. What's more is that both the walking and drinking water could be done anywhere I travelled. I didn't really need a gym at that point; I just needed to keep moving and drinking water!

It was the happiest case of "accidental success" I had ever experienced!

What's Eating You?

In any situation life throws at us, it is important to know what to do, which can sometimes be defined by what *not* to do! If you are going to buy a car or a home, you would, no doubt, do some research ahead of time. I encourage you to do the same when it comes to what you are going to be putting into your body and the body of your child. You wouldn't put turpentine into your car now, would you? The same applies for what you put into your body's "fuel tank."

LABELS

When we shop for food, we are bombarded by terms on packages that tout the health benefits of a particular product. A word to the wise, these terms often may mean something different than what we understand them to mean. In fact, some of what is being packaged as being "good for you" may not be very good for us at all.

Here are some pitfalls and cautionary points that can help you steer clear of trouble and disappointment.

"Diet Foods"

Forget them. They do not exist. There is no magic food with pixie dust powers that will melt fat off your body. All there is is *real* food and how you eat it, in conjunction with a healthy lifestyle.

Trans Fats and Hydrogenated Oils

Avoid this like the plague. It is a man-made substance created for the preservation of "food" and "enriched" taste. In short, you take a stick of butter, add some oil, blast it together with hydrogen and then add bleach along with a metal agent to keep it all together. *Voila!* Trans fat! Check labels for anything hydrogenated, such as hydrogenated soybean oil, palm kernel oils etc. Chances are the cookies, frozen pancakes and yes, even the diet food items you may have in your home, may contain at least some of these. Your body has no clue what to do with a trans fat. Why? Well it is not a natural substance and the year after it was invented and hit the markets, America found itself with the first cases of coronary disease. Coronary diseases simply did not exist until trans fats arrived. It can separate your fat genes, reorganize them and create new ones that your body has no clue what to do with, and among other things, cause adult onset diabetes and in some cases, even cancer. Do you really want to be eating that stuff?

"HFCS" (High Fructose Corn Syrup).
Many times sweeter than actual raw sugar and a fraction of the cost to produce and re-sell. Nearly all pop is loaded with it, as well as candy. At the movie theater when you order your favourite soft drink, be prepared to take in the equivalent of up to a whopping 12 tablespoons of sugar! Yummy!

"Lose ten lb. in two weeks," etc. types of promises and diets.
Sure, starvation will get you to lose weight, but it will never last. Why? Simply because there is no way on earth you could eat like that for the rest of your life. Diets such as these merely restrict caloric intake. I could write a diet based entirely on eating potato chips. Would you lose weight? Of course you would. Would it be healthy for you? Of course not. All that would happen is that your body would experience a dramatic drop in the calories you are taking in and you would lose weight, but your cholesterol would jump sky high, which is nothing to say of the precious lean muscle tissue you would cannibalize as well! The moment you go back to a higher caloric intake, all the weight you lost (primarily muscle and water) would come right back.

FOOD TERMS AND SO CALLED "HEALTHY LABELING"

Remember, the food industry is in business for profit. Since the competition for your dollars is fierce, advertisers will do anything possible to lure you to their product. Some of the terms to watch for are as follows:

"**Enriched**"- this really means that the natural state of the product has been messed with by man. Originally, to "enrich" a food product meant to add certain vitamins and minerals, not a bad thing. Unfortunately, it also brought about the addition of sugars and bleach in most cases, and it also means that whatever was in the food in the first place which was good for you has been either compromised, extracted, or eliminated entirely. God got food right the first time, man does not need to "enrich" or improve upon what is already perfect. Stick to the naturals!

"Made with...100% real fruit juice" (or some other product using similar terminology).

If I make a fruit juice product to sell on the market and I make it with 90% sugar and preservatives and include 10% actual fruit juice, I am in a position to legally say it was made with *real* fruit juice. Clever, isn't it?

"Contains no added MSG, sugar, fat," etc.

It might mean that there is a *ton* of the stuff in there already that is not good for you. The fact that they did not add to the bad stuff is pretty irrelevant. It's just on the label as an advertisement to get you to pick up the product and to make think that it's good for you.

"A low source of fat or carbs," etc.

Terrific; so what? What about the salt or sugar levels and the cholesterol bombs the product may contain? Once again, this is to lure your attention off of the questionable ingredients in the product and aim your focus towards the "good" things. Also, if you do not eat carbs at all, you are in for a whack of trouble. The instant you come off a no/low carb diet, the second your body even sniffs a carb it will hang onto it for dear life. Is that realistic? Can you really eat like that for your entire life?

REMEMBER: The food industry is in this for profit. Like a car manufacturer, they advertise for your dollar. It is their right to do so since profit is the reason they went into business in the first place. Don't fall for it! There are some *very* good food companies out there producing healthy foods.

Just do your research and get educated!

Yesterday, Malnutrition Seemed So Far Away

We Italians love to eat. I often jokingly tell my clients that "we invented eating!" Our cuisine is as fundamental a part of our culture as Michelangelo, the Pope, Ferrari, and gli Azzurri (our nation's soccer team).

Therefore, let me shout this from the mountain tops: I EAT CARBS. I LIKE CARBS and YOU, gentle reader, SHOULD also eat carbs!

Let's have a look at the Romans back around the time of Caesar Augustus. What were these people eating back then?

A typical Roman diet:

- *carrots, onions, radishes, celery, polenta (cornbread), lentils, centaury, mushrooms, truffles, flax seeds, chick peas, broad beans, spinach, lettuce (watercress, chicory, endive, leek leaves), artichokes, asparagus*
- *figs, olives, apples, plums, pears, cherries, dates, quinces, grapes*
- *nuts: hazelnuts, pistachios, chestnuts, pine nuts, walnuts and almonds*
- *sole, sea bass, sturgeon, tuna, whiting fish and red mullet, sharks, whales, sardines, anchovies, gilthead, etc.*
- *lobster, crabs, shrimp, prawns, sea urchins, squid, cuttlefish, octopus, oysters, clams, carp, trout, salmon, kid, lamb, mutton, veal, beef, pork, hare, rabbit, guinea fowl, chickens and capons, goose, ducks, pigeons, turkeys and pheasant, deer, gazelle, goat, hare, rabbit*
- *eggs, cheeses, milk (sheep, goat, cow)*
- *spices and seasonings: juniper, dill, onion, saffron, mint, fen-*

nel, mustard, cumin, oil, vinegar, garum (a fermented fish paste), honey, salt and lard
- wheat, oats (that's bread), whole grains (not "enriched")

Wow, I'm getting full just *looking* at that list!

Okay, granted, there are some foods mentioned above that we don't hear much of these days, but we are all familiar with the majority of the other items.

Notice anything? I sure do. *Tons* of foods, no brand names, no gimmicks, and it all came from the earth. This food was all there before large chain supermarkets, packaging, or fast food eateries existed, In fact, it has been in existence as long as man himself! Why did we stray? Why the potato chips, the diet sodas, the low carb, the "diet" foods now? WHY? Were these food inventions really necessary?

LET'S GET BACK TO THE ROOTS, folks! The answer to healthy living has been here forever!

Ancient Roman people were fit and they walked nearly everywhere. Do we think that those mighty gladiators and warriors chowed down on "protein bars" or pumped steroids?

Imagine telling an Italian that he *cannot* eat bread, pizza or pasta. Imagine telling a Mexican or a Greek person that he cannot eat pita. Imagine telling a Frenchman he can't have that crusty French roll. Now imagine yourself running away from all of those wonderful people as fast as you can, 'cause you will *need* to, should you choose to utter such nonsense! (Hey, at least you're *running*. It's good exercise!)

THOSE FAMOUS DIETS WE HAVE ALL HEARD OF

The second a "diet" program requires you to delete a food group altogether, is the second it becomes unhealthy and unrealistic. (Unless of course, you are allergic to certain foods.) The second a diet requires you to weigh everything you eat and count every calorie, fat, protein, and carbohydrate gram is the second it becomes unmanageable. The second a diet program sells you *their special food*, is the same instant you realize that it becomes expensive and unrealistic. What happens when you find yourself at a party or on vacation and you cannot get to your "special diet" food? It's GAME OVER, or rather, over-weight!

Here it is in very plain terms. A diet plan wants to sell you its own brand of "diet" food because they are banking on the fact that you are uneducated and incapable of figuring out what to eat on your own. To tell you the truth, it borders on insulting, however, "ignorance is expensive."

No "magic food" exists, but the food that the Romans ate and the food God put on the earth *does exist*. Just who are these "brilliant engineers" who have devised food that supposedly helps you to lose weight? If such food existed I would know about it and I would have used it. Actually, in my research, I did try a host of "diet" foods and bars. Know what? They tasted awful and some of them were so high in calories that I may as well have gotten myself a *real* chocolate bar at the variety store! "Simulated chocolate" or "chocolate substitute"? Forget it! There is *no* substitute for chocolate. It is glorious! How about we just eat real chocolate instead? Wow, what a concept! Of course, it has to be *in moderation*, but give me the real stuff!

Would it surprise you to know that most of the leading frozen "diet food" in the freezer section at your local supermarket, as well as so called "health" or "power bars," contain those two horrendous ingredients I listed in my chapter entitled, "What's Eating You?"—HFCS and Trans fat? Is that not the apex of hypocrisy?

The only reason these frozen "diet foods" *might* work has nothing to do with the ingredients or the food; some of them are downright bad for you. It does, however, have everything to do with "portion control." Guess what? YOU can achieve portion control all on your own *without* paying an exorbitant amount of money and without the killer ingredients. Again, these companies are telling you, "hey, you are too lazy and ignorant to know how *not* to eat 5,000 calories in one meal, so here, we'll do it for you. Now just hand over your wallet!"

In essence, what has happened to a lot of the "diet (health) food" industry is exactly the same concept of drive-through junk food. A disclaimer here, I do believe that SOME of these prepackaged "health foods" are better for you than junk food.

INSTANT SOCIETY

Having said that, both the frozen diet food and junk fast food industries have a few things in common:

Both play into the idea of an "instant society." By way of this, they both fuel the concept that you have no time to cook or sit and eat. The breakdown of social structures and families is a whole other subject worth writing a few thousand books about!

By making the "food" easily accessible, they, in a sense, are able to "dictate" what you will eat. You can stop this influence on your life, of course, by taking control of your own food plan and schedule. Like any habit, good or bad, this will take time to form, but you have to start by at least making an effort.

They both figure you *trust them* to feed you something that is nutritious, or that you are too ignorant to figure out what *is* and what *isn't* healthy on your own.

Both of those industries make billions upon billions of dollars, thanks to people who subscribe to their points of view.

"Instant" is big business.

Burgers, fries, chips, tacos, donuts, muffins, shakes, ice cream, hot dogs, canned soda pop, calorie laden "designer" coffees and candy bars...all of these are "instant." Pop into a convenience store or drive-through at 4 a.m. and you'll find these readily available.

"Instant" is indeed convenient and even I like instant.

I hear you out there: *Hey dude, I am on-the-go constantly, I NEED instant. INSTANT is good. I do not have time to cook, much less sit and eat for that matter.*

(Warning! The next paragraph is going to challenge you to radically change your way of thinking and also has the potential to save your life.)

FRUITS, VEGETABLES, AND WHOLE GRAINS are also INSTANT!

Ta-Daa!

Yes, all of the stuff that is good for us is also readily available, but is rare, if not impossible to find at a drive-through. WHY? Well, because healthy food will spoil and go bad and it also has a short "shelf life." Know what? It's supposed to spoil and eventually die Real food is "alive," just like you are!

IT IS UP TO YOU TO TAKE CONTROL!

Get a Ziplock bag and put good things in it to eat in the car. Stop for a sub meal combo? That's about ten dollars where I live. Know how much fresh and real food ten bucks can buy? At *least* four days' worth! While you're at it, keep a case of water bottles in the car. An entire case of 24 bottles of the life giving stuff costs about $4! One *can* of the stuff that poisons you costs about half as much, and water also has *no* calories. AMAZING!

What's that you say? You don't like water? How about you add something to it such as lemon or maybe lime?

In my chapter "Starving to be Fat," you read about stored energy. Water works in much the same way. If you do not drink enough of it, your body will go into a dehydrated state (without you even feeling thirsty) and will store all the water already in your system for as long as it can. You could be carrying over 10 lb. of "water weight!"

We need to hydrate! What happens to a plant if you do not water it? Get the idea?

Implement your re-hydration plan gradually over time. If you barely have a glass of water a day as a way of life right now, and you all of the sudden take in litres of it, you are going to spend all night in the bathroom. Make sure you keep a copy of my book in there! If, instead, you initially choose to add even one glass per day, the chances of it finally becoming a habit are greatly increased. People who are not used to drinking water will develop a distaste (though water is tasteless) for it and as a result will feel overwhelmed and may give up on the practice entirely.

All I can say is GO SLOW at first and think long term. Pick up a copy of "the Tortoise and the Hare," it's a great example.

Trainers
Certified or Certifiable?

Ever had a chance to get irritated at someone driving on the road? They cut you off, hand signals are exchanged, etc. Oh, come on now! Am I the only one that is vehicularly challenged?

Know what is even more frightening about "those other" drivers? They all have a licence! They passed a test and are certified to drive. But wow, what do they drive like?

A "certified" trainer, can unfortunately be as inept as many of those drivers. Passing an exam, for example the bar exam to become a lawyer, does not mean you are a good lawyer, it means you studied to pass a test. What makes a trainer great is what he or she does both up to and following that certification.

The sexiest looking car in the lot, may not be the best car for you.

Just because a trainer looks incredible, does not mean they have the knowledge to train *you*!

Now, I want to be very careful to not broad stroke every trainer on earth as being incompetent, since that is certainly not the case. I have worked with hundreds of personal trainers and I must say, there are some who are simply brilliant! Then again, there are some who really should stick to only training themselves!

WHAT TO LOOK FOR IN A TRAINER

While taking my previous paragraph into balanced consideration, you should absolutely make sure the trainer has at least the most basic qualifications and is accredited by a reputable governing fitness body.

If you are considering hiring a trainer, go to a gym and watch the trainers on the floor for at least a week. You should do this to see what their work ethic is like with their existing clients. You will usually find that the same trainers usually stand out. These are the ones who are evidently and actively involved with their clients.

The Major Red Flags!

- Trainer has arms crossed and is not physically engaging the client, nor spotting/guiding them.
- Trainer is on cell phone, during the session.
- Trainer is consistently late and does not make up for clients' lost time.
- Trainer is looking at the ceiling or the cute blonde when attention should be focused on their client.
- Trainer is eating fried chicken during the session. (Yes, I have actually seen this!)

A "personal" trainer, should be both personal in their dealings with you, as well as personable. The character fit has to be there or there will be no chemistry and you will both find it hard to communicate and get results. Different personalities respond to a variety of stimuli. Some respond to being softly encouraged, while others prefer the "drill sergeant" mentality. There is no shortage of personalities and again, it would be a good idea for you to watch a trainer on the gym floor and see how they interact with their clients. Integrity is what takes place when someone does the right thing, even when they are not aware they are being watched.

Inquire at the gym as to what the trainer's client retention is, also known as his/her renewal rate. If a trainer retains his clients, that is almost a sure sign that the clients are happy with the trainer and are seeing results.

Talk to one or two of the trainer's clients and ask them how their experience has been so far. The client will always tell you the truth about how their investment has paid out.

TRAINING A BEGINNER

If you are overweight and you have been inactive, or have only been doing cardio for years, DO NOT split the body when starting weight workouts. Do NOT listen to a trainer who tells you to do so. By way of simple example; your first sessions with a trainer should not focus solely on arms, legs, abs, etc. You are in a deconditioned state and a foundation must first be built and developed. At first, the entire body must be worked. If you begin to load (put free or machine weight on) only one body part, the risk for injury and imbalances will greatly increase. If your trainer is a bodybuilder type, he or she may insist on splitting the body immediately and I can tell you that is not the way to go at first.

What you should be looking at is cross training or circuit training. These involve major muscle groups and the workouts are designed to be non stop. Believe me, you will feel like you ran at high intensity for half an hour, if these training principles are properly executed. You will reap double the benefits by building muscle AND burning fat.

WHAT TO "BUY"

Trainers are not cheap, so you should make sure you are getting the best bang for your buck. Here are a few simple ways to get the most out of your personal training experience.

Do not waste your money by buying one session in hopes that it will solve your challenges. Invest as much as you can in your health, it should be your top priority. It is impossible for even Arnold Schwarzenegger to tell you how to get it all done in one hour.

If you can afford to work with a trainer once per week, no matter how little or much you can afford, make absolutely sure that the trainer will write you a program to follow on days when you are training alone. This is VITAL! You cannot be in a position of making progress only when you are working with a trainer, and since most people can't afford a trainer three times per week, get mileage, get a program.

Whatever program you receive from your trainer must evolve. This is to prevent your body from hitting a plateau and no longer making progress. The human body is incredibly adaptive! It can survive in blazing heat or arctic conditions, with food or without etc. In the same way, it will quickly adapt to whatever you are doing and work to keep you there.

If you can't afford very much, make sure to at least get something to get you started, but beware. Suppose you purchase eight personal training sessions in a package (most gyms sell training in this fashion), do NOT fall into the trap of using them all up in one month. Here is why: once you have made some initial progress, if your sessions run out, you will basically be stuck because you will not know what to do from that point forward. Simplest example? You start at 38% body fat and a certain weight. You work with a pro, rip through all of your sessions, lose eight lb. and your body fat drops to 35% initially. Great! Now what? A person who decreases body fat, even slightly and loses a few lb., cannot train in the same fashion as where they began. The body has changed, and therefore the workout must change to cause constant progression at this new and healthier stage.

Remember this: A "routine" can't do it for you. It must change as your body changes and your body will not change unless the program changes.

COMMUNICATE!

There is pain associated with muscle growth, and if you have been inactive, you may also suffer from creaky bones, joints etc.

If there is acute pain (sudden and sharp) during an exercise, I don't care if you are training with Rambo, STOP IMMEDIATELY! Especially us guys, we are horrible for this, since we think we can push through anything. Even though it might be possible to indeed push through that pain, it does not mean you should! Talk to your trainer and tell them what is going on. Muscular training pain is different than trauma and it must be addressed immediately. Disclose any and all injuries, as well as your medical conditions, both past and present. Don't be a hero by not telling your trainer about "that chest pain I had a year ago, but it was nothing," because you can wind up being a dead hero, and the world already has enough of those! Before even getting near a gym floor, your trainer should have had you fill out a PAR-Q type of form. This stands for Physical Activity Readiness Questionnaire. In this document, all information should be recorded and given to your trainer for conversation and follow up.

GET A GOOD NUTRITIONIST!

Experts agree that successful and permanent weight loss is largely accredited to proper, healthy, and balanced eating. In fact, those same experts agree that proper nutrition is at least 70% responsible for achieving permanent weight loss. Do not ask your trainer for nutrition advice, as this is a completely different discipline. Some trainers know what works for them, but it does not mean it will necessarily work for you as well.

Do *not* work with a nutritionist who will try to put you on a "diet." What you should look for is a professional who can educate you and provide you with a written meal plan that is based on real food, not supplements (though these have their place) or protein bars and fad foods. If you work with a nutritionist who asks you to eliminate an entire food group forever, be it carbs or fats, rest assured you will be destined and doomed to fail. Restriction diets work for a while, but are they truly manageable for life, or even healthy? If you are a sales professional who travels a lot and lives out of a suitcase, it is going to be very difficult if not impossible for you to plan meals and cook them ahead of time. A competent nutritionist should see this and, in turn, write a meal plan that teaches you what the wisest choices in a restaurant or board room might be. Your eating plan must be "real life" and manageable, no matter where you find yourself.

Yes, there may be extreme cases when a doctor will consult with a nutritionist and, in certain cases, you may be advised to temporarily follow a prescribed diet for medical reasons. Please be cautious should you ever receive such advice. I am not saying it may not be correct given a particular situation, but doctors are not nutritionists and most nutritionists are not doctors. Yes, there are always exceptions, but to find a professional who is also competent in both fields is in fact not the norm.

Referrals are another way of finding a reputable trainer or nutritionist. I know that if I am looking for a mechanic, plumber or anything of the sort, that I will probably ask a trusted friend if they know of anyone in the field. Research your trainer, just as you would research a car purchase by finding out all you can in advance. You may even ask the gym (or trainer) for a trial session, agreeing to pay for the service if the trainer is right for you.

No one is perfect, but there *is* a trainer out there who is perfect for you.

DO I REALLY NEED A TRAINER?

My first trainer basically saved my life and set me on a course that got me to where I am, but the rest was up to me. How important do I think a good personal trainer, nutritionist and programs from both are to your success? Well, to put it quite simply, I am a certified trainer with a history of satisfied clients and yet I still hire a personal trainer and nutritionist to keep me on track and always challenge me.

Perhaps you could start your search by visiting your local gym nearby and "spying out the land," to see who on the gym floor looks like they could help you change your life.

With the right trainer and nutritionist, I can pretty much promise you that this will be the best investment you will ever make!

Final Thoughts

Thank you for taking the time to read my book. I hope it has at least served to help you in starting or continuing your fitness journey. Please don't think that everyday is easy for me. Even now, after all my weight loss progress to date, there are still days when I struggle to get myself into the gym and train. I still deal with everyday pressures of life just as many of you do. I do know that even when I have to force myself to get into the gym that I always feel better after I have completed my workout. Some workouts go better than others. There are days when I feel I nailed it, and then there are what Susan and I both call "dragfests," better than nothing workouts.

Even now, when I look in the mirror, I struggle with body image and often feel my progress is never quite good enough. That's the time when I must remind myself of how far I have come and what I felt like on that very first day so many years ago, when I got on a treadmill and had the most embarrassing experience of my life.

Do not pay attention to anyone who may ridicule you, or tell you that you will never succeed. The most successful people in history were the ones who most often faced staggering opposition and ridicule. Most of all, do this for YOU and no one else. Yes, it may benefit your marriage and keep you around longer for your children, all of which are wonderful by-products of you making these positive changes, however, you must do this as an act of love for yourself.

If you have a bad day, a bad week, do NOT quit. NEVER give up. Remember that failure is only defined as such when you make a conscious declaration that you have failed. It does not matter how many times you try, you must keep going. Thomas Edison made over 10,000 attempts before successfully inventing the lightbulb. Here is what he had to say on the matter : "Nearly every man who develops an idea works at it up to the point where it looks impossible, and then gets discouraged. That's not the place to become discouraged."

The good news for you is that this book has provided you with a guideline on how to greatly improve the chances for your success. Remember, it was not written by a historian or a researcher, it was written by a person who has accomplished what less than 3 percent of the population has: I've lost well over 100 lb. and have kept it off. In fact continued to lose for nearly a decade. I tell you this not to make myself seem haughty, but to instead hopefully inspire you as only a person who has accomplished this can.

Don't starve to be fat any longer. Instead, starve your fat and your defeat by feeding yourself with positive action.

May God's richest blessings find you and completely overtake you. See you on the speaking circuit.

Marco

For more information, please visit me on line at : www.wiredtowin.ca

Info@marcogs.com

www.wiredtowin.ca